SECOND EDITION

SIMPLE

The Inner Game of Ophthalmic Practice Success

SECOND EDITION

SIMPLE

The Inner Game of Ophthalmic Practice Success

John B. Pinto

CRC Press
Taylor & Francis Group
Boca Raton London New York

CRC Press is an imprint of the
Taylor & Francis Group, an **informa** business

John B. Pinto *is an ophthalmology practice management consultant in his firm, J. Pinto & Associates, Inc.* Dr. Richard L. Lindstrom *has not disclosed any relevant financial relationships.* Dr. Craig N. Piso *has no financial or proprietary interest in the materials presented herein.*

First published 2008 by SLACK Incorporated

Published 2024 by CRC Press
2385 NW Executive Center Drive, Suite 320, Boca Raton FL 33431

and by CRC Press
4 Park Square, Milton Park, Abingdon, Oxon, OX14 4RN

CRC Press is an imprint of Taylor & Francis Group, LLC

Library of Congress Control Number: 2021941150

Cover Artist: Lori Shields

ISBN: 9781630919597 (pbk)
ISBN: 9781003526414 (ebk)

DOI: 10.1201/9781003526414

SIMPLE
Syml
Bakar
بسيط
Eenvoudige
Senp
সহজ
Yksinkertainen
簡單
Simpleng
פשוט
Yooj yim
Простой
Egyszerű
Απλο
Basit
애 인
Sencillo
シンプル
Preprosta
Einfa

DEDICATION

This book is dedicated with affection to the world's roughly 50,000 ophthalmic practices … and their respective 200,000 ophthalmologists, million-plus support staff, and seven billion potential patients.

My deepest gratitude for allowing me the opportunity, over the last 40 years and all the years remaining, to simultaneously be a student and a teacher within this elegant, confounding, evolving, and marvelously deep profession.

Contents

Acknowledgments

To My Teachers
Mom and Dad and Sister Laura
Miss Short
A Four-Inch Rainbow Trout
Mr. Hassan
Camp Fox and the Midnight Cot Caper
Grant Neely
Boyd Smith
Osiris
Julie R.
Sierra Nevada
Hemingway
Mescalito
Paul Saltman
Bob Holly
Henry David Thoreau
The First Third of El Capitan
Gibran
Big Al Kildow
Jonas Salk
Francis Crick
Paris
Madame Atger and Jean-Philippe
S/V Chrysalis
Sir Francis Bacon
The Pacific Ocean
E. F. Schumacher
Samantha
Jim Rohn
Doug Simay
David Schneider … and belatedly, golf
John "Ain't Done Crashin' Yet" Corboy
Whitney and Graham
Lucy Santiago
Michel Arowns, Martine Cartier et Familles
Dick Lindstrom's Generous Mind and Cellar
The Crane Meadow Lodge Follies
Rioja in Boston
Craig Piso's Healthy Power
The Black Beast
The Zafu
The Ukulele
And Mom … again

About the Author

"Life Is Only Teaching and Learning."

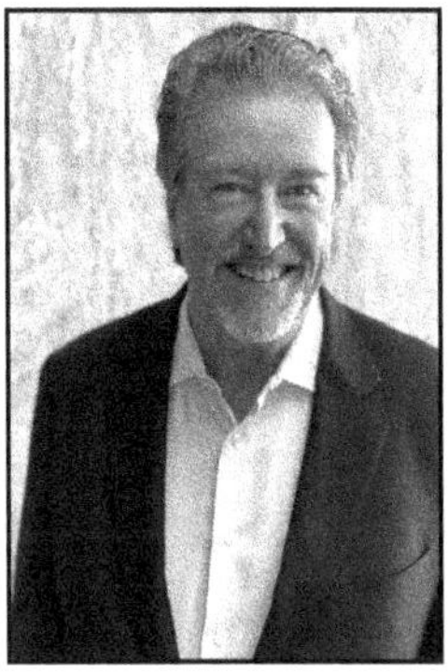

John B. Pinto is the most-published author in America on ophthalmology practice management topics. He founded J. Pinto & Associates, Inc, an ophthalmic practice management consulting firm, in 1979. Since then he has provided strategic planning, operations, and marketing advice to pharmaceutical companies, basic science centers, hospitals, multispecialty clinics, and single-specialty facilities.

For over 40 years, a majority of the firm's service has been to ophthalmic practices ranging from small solo practices to high-volume market leaders, teaching centers, and ophthalmic product companies. He has been active as a practice consultant in North America and Europe, and has worked and lectured in South America and the Far East.

Pinto is best known as a strategic planning and economic advisor to practices large and small. In addition to covering most dimensions of modern practice operations management, he is a career advisor—providing individual coaching and contract negotiation services to new graduates and midcareer ophthalmologists. His professional life today is rounded out with succession planning, practice valuations, partner dispute mediation, merger/acquisition counsel, and leadership development for administrators and physicians.

A prolific writer, Pinto is the author of several books beyond the text you now hold:

- *John Pinto's Little Green Book of Ophthalmology*
- *Turnaround: Twenty-One Weeks to Ophthalmic Practice Survival and Permanent Improvement*
- *Ten Eyecare Practices: Benchmarks for Success*
- *Cash Flow: The Practical Art of Earning More From Your Ophthalmology Practice,* written with Anne Rose
- *The Efficient Ophthalmologist*
- *Legal Issues in Ophthalmology: A Review for Surgeons and Administrators,* written with Alan Reider and Allison Shuren
- *The Women of Ophthalmology,* written with Elizabeth Davis, MD
- *Ophthalmic Leadership: A Practical Guide for Physicians, Administrators, and Teams*
- *Marketing Your Ophthalmic Practice*

Many of these titles are now published and can be ordered by going to www.routledge.com.

John is a member of the editorial board of *Ocular Surgery News* and a regular contributor to other eye care publications. He is available for individual physician and practice consulting services to supplement this book. Please contact him at:

J. Pinto & Associates, Inc.
2926 Kellogg Street Suite B18
San Diego, CA 92106
619-223-2233
pintoinc@aol.com
www.pintoinc.com

Foreword

Choose the life that is most useful,
and habit will make it the most agreeable.
—Sir Francis Bacon

As ophthalmologists, we are experts at complexity. We excel at minutia. We parse and re-parse the smallest details.

That's great for our patients, and terrific intellectually, but sometimes it's not so great for our medical practices—where seeing the big picture and keeping things simple is the key to business success.

For most of 4 decades, John Pinto, our profession's "ophthalmologist-ologist" and leading advisor, has studied our strengths and our weaknesses and helped an international community of surgeons deal with our ever-growing business and organizational challenges.

This new book, *Simple,* is exactly that. Whether you are in the first or the last 5 years of your career as an ophthalmologist, the maxims and truths in this book will help you be more successful.

John has distilled some 50,000 hours of on-site consulting work throughout America and the world into those factors and professional habits which—once mastered—will decrease the frustrations and uncertainties felt by all of us as practice owners and leaders.

—Richard L. Lindstrom, MD
Minnesota Eye Consultants
Minneapolis, Minnesota

Introduction

A prudent question is one-half of wisdom.

—Sir Francis Bacon

Of Reality

Ophthalmology may be an elegant profession, but it is not in the least simple. Eye care practitioners are wicked-smart. They have a tolerance for—and more than that, are drawn to—things that are complex. Why else would a procedure like cataract surgery with essentially perfect outcomes since the turn of the century still be such an active sphere of ongoing innovation and elaboration?

These intellectually gratifying clinical and surgical complexities (that at least stand to marginally improve patient outcomes) are unfortunately matched by galloping complexities that won't add value to patients in the years ahead:

- Coding and documentation changes take time away from patient care (and caring), and the chase to document meaningful use is probably shortening administrator lifespans.
- Local hospital-provider consolidation and competitive encroachment threaten the independence of nearly every private practice in America today.
- Third-party payer reform included under the Affordable Care Act is making everyone a bit crazy and a lot insecure.

As unaccustomed as it is in ophthalmology, "simple" is at least a partial antidote for everything that makes ophthalmic practice so vexing. "Simple" mitigates (to some degree) a world of increasing elaboration. Simplicity includes the following:

- Taking pride in the smallest and most time-and-motion-efficient office facilities you can get by with, instead of the largest facilities you can afford
- Employing a small, long-tenured, crack team of cross-trained support staff rather than a fleet of newbies
- Eliminating all patient services and conversations that do not add value
- Getting physically fit and mentally clear enough to breeze through the extra patients needed to sustain practice cash flow as fees stagnate
- Providing such great customer service that external marketing is no longer needed
- Simplifying call coverage to every possible degree
- Wearing scrubs to reduce costs while increasing professional appearance
- Removing all the clutter from your office space
- Arranging simple appointment templates with shorts and longs, rather than fractionating into a dozen or more appointment types that nobody at the front desk can keep straight
- Avoiding expensive trips down the rabbit hole to try out yet another "sure-fire" practice adjunct (read: facial skin resurfacing, hair removal, medi-spas, hearing aid centers, and the like)
- Working 40 hours a week in 4 days instead of 5
- Taking the office paperless all the way, not only for electronic health records

- Making time to enjoy a midday run, lunch out, or that long-lost escape to the golf course on Wednesday afternoon
- Living closer to your office to save commuting time
- Changing your personal lifestyle so that you own your practice instead of your practice owning you

• • •

As a management consultant, I am a curator of practical things that work. Of necessity, I ignore much of that which is new and fashionable and exciting.

Most new business ideas, like most first thoughts in science and medicine and politics and architecture, are bunkum. We humans, in the main, are an unwise species. Baked in the cake is a predilection to ignore data, avoid difficult conversations, and follow imprudent leaders. This happens as much within the smallest ophthalmology practice as it does in the broader world.

Here in Eyeland, we have all been happily habituated to relative stability, both as citizens of a nation at the top of the heap since the end of World War II and as participants in the prosperous field of ophthalmology. This is not likely to last.

Our accustomed, affluent status quo is doomed for myriad reasons—the competitive rise of the rest of the world, political fatigue in the industrial West, erratic but generally rising energy costs, the accelerating substitution of technology for human labor, a natural pullback in the US economy as boomers retire, and the long-recognized reality that we have vastly overshot the mark on what can be affordably spent as a nation on health care services.

And that is before even considering the galloping pace at which private specialty practices will be absorbed into deep-pocketed regional health systems, with much of the profession's accustomed ancillary profits being shifted to institutional bottom lines.

The era of ophthalmic affluence will pass for all but the most entrepreneurial providers. These few physicians are now climbing up the industrial curve by employing many associate doctors or developing technologies to provide more care with fewer resources. Your personal ophthalmic income will still be based on your personal merit and work intensity, but the ophthalmic baseline income of the future will be somewhat lower than it is today.

It is not all that bad. In the future, most ophthalmologists will still be compensated at levels somewhat higher than the wages enjoyed by other intelligent knowledge workers: PhD historians, nuclear physicists, entomologists, and the like. These individuals are as brilliant as you and have learned to be as fulfilled as you are today, but in ways that are more economical. While they are underpaid in the context of their brains, dedication, and training—as you will one day be—they have survived, as will all of those ophthalmologists-to-be who are now preschoolers as this book goes to press.

As gruesome as this may sound for you (and your young children now bound for medical school), it is nothing like what's in store for the roughly 40% of American workers today who will become a permanent underclass when their jobs are offshored or automated. The growing 1% vs 99% inequality we are seeing today is just a foretaste of what's to come, when workers will cleave into those who are good at building and working with intelligent machines, and those who will be replaced by machines.

All the technology that is needed to replace the cognitive dimension of medical eye care—branching logic trees, algorithms, and the rest—is readily available today. Robot ophthalmic diagnostics just is not here yet because the market is too small compared to other interesting segments of the economy, like automated stock trading. But soon enough, artificial intelligence will shrink the market value of squishy human ophthalmologist brains.

Most of the data inputs needed to work up a patient (eg, history, vision, pressure, images) are already gathered by machines and technicians. We are not far off from a day when the suspected diagnosis and prospective treatment plan is already on the monitor when you first enter a new patient's exam room, just awaiting your confirmation or revision.

Of course, that delicious, profoundly gratifying, manual, surgical dimension of ophthalmology will remain human-dependent for many more years. But not forever. Cataract surgery is now so routine and present in such industrially high volumes, and increasingly machine-assisted, that it will yield soon enough (and perhaps before many other surgeries) to labor substitution by dexterous, clever, machine-guided technicians.

Along the way, we are likely to see some very unaccustomed permutations on how eye care is delivered. Homeowners now use internet listings to rent out overnight rooms to strangers, and private car owners are now running app-based cab services. Is it impossible to imagine an era when some underemployed ophthalmologists and optometrists start making house calls or seeing patients for cash in a converted spare bedroom?

• • •

Much of what follows in this book is aimed not at any ultimate solution to what's coming over the long-term horizon, but at helping you accommodate and make the best of the changes as they slowly unfurl. So it goes.

• • •

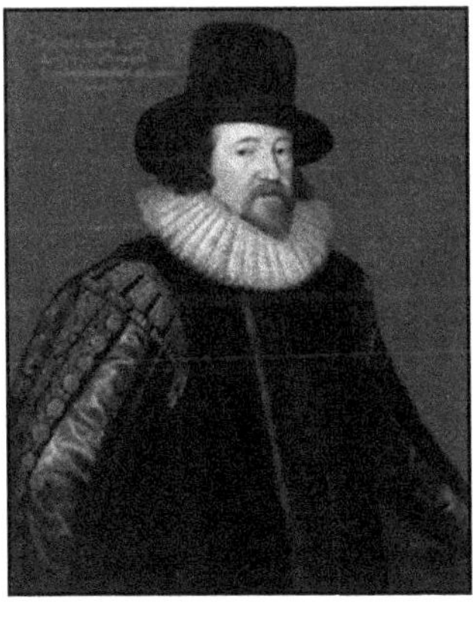

The structure of this book is adopted from that of a much earlier, and much wiser, advisor and writer, Sir Francis Bacon. Bacon was an English philosopher, scientist, and essayist. In late 16th-century England, he first wrote and later improved a series of short instructions called *Essays.* With titles like "Of Cunning" and "Of Beauty," this book became a guide for living and prospering in 17th-century Europe.

Nearly 4 centuries later, I first read Bacon's *Essays* in the South of France at the age of 25. I was naïvely and madly in love, pursuing (completely without result) the daughter of a senior United Nations official. Bacon was a great comfort to me then in my unrequited state.

There are but two tragedies in life. One is one's inability to attain one's heart's desire. The other is to have it.

—Sir Francis Bacon

Today, nearly 4 decades on, Bacon is still a comfort and, in retrospect, an intellectual touchstone for much of my work. Each of the short pieces in this book are similarly titled as the essays in Bacon's great work. "Of Cunning" and "Of Beauty" are absent, but in their place you will find subjects like, "Of Partnership" and "Of Adaptability."

I harbor no expectations that this short book will be read in the centuries ahead. But I hope you find it a useful guide to transiting the challenges of the present day.

—John B. Pinto
San Diego, California

CHAPTER 1

Testing Your Practice on Twenty-Five Simple Things

If a man will begin with certainties, he shall end in doubts; but if he will be content to begin with doubts, he shall end in certainties.
—Sir Francis Bacon

Ophthalmology is a maddeningly complex and precise enterprise relative to its comparatively small financial scale. The former head of operations of a $2 billion engineering firm, who took on responsibility for running a $55 million eye clinic, once remarked to me, "This practice is more difficult to run than a multinational company many times this size."

Pablo Picasso once said, "I am always doing that which I cannot do, in order that I may learn how to do it." He was obviously on to something. Although estimates vary, it is believed that Mr. Picasso produced more than 50,000 discrete works of art, including paintings, sculptures, ceramics, and prints. And that's before counting his lesser-known poetry and plays.

Pinto JB. *Simple: The Inner Game of Ophthalmic Practice Success, Second Edition* (pp 1-4).

Keep trying, trying. At the end of the day, practice success boils down to doing just 25 simple things well, over and over again.

But, as a surgeon you will do Picasso one better. In your own career, you'll probably knock out about 180,000 works of art, including all patient encounters and all surgical cases. And then there's that piece of art (although some would use other words) called "your professional practice." It, too, for all its lumps and warts, is also your personal creation. It, too, deserves efforts at constant improvement and attempts to do the difficult thing.

To find out how well you and your staff are doing at managing the business side of your profession, I've created a simple self-test. Below you'll find 25 key hallmarks of practice success. There could as easily be 50 or 100, but after years of fieldwork, I think that these 25 are the most important.

Read through each one and then score your practice—and your board and management team—on the following scale:

4 We've nailed it—we do this, and do it well!
3 We do this, but could probably make improvements.
2 We do this on and off, but not well or consistently.
1 We have done this in the past, but not for some time.
0 We have never done this.

____ 1. *A written strategic plan*—that completely describes, with appropriate time horizons, the mission and values, the intended service area, growth rate, service and provider mix, positioning strategy, and alignment with other market participants. Used as an active document, it provides the context for tactical priorities.

____ 2. *Written tactical priorities*—driven by the strategic plan and limited at any one time to a realistically accomplishable list of near-term actions and objectives.

____ 3. *Administrator/executive director (ED)/CEO*—of appropriate experience, skill, and time commitment whose competencies are aligned with the practice's current needs. The appropriate mix of leadership/executive vs management/operations talent for the scale of the practice. An appropriate balance between "hard" skills (eg, finance, accounting, regulatory, product knowledge) and "soft" skills (eg, human resources, communication, conflict resolution, marketing); rewards are proportionate to performance and aligned with the owners.

____ 4. *Managing partner (MP)*—an inspirational group leader, who is selected based on (a) the current needs of the practice, (b) the candidate's skill, and (c) the candidate's desire to lead. A 2+ year tenure with no term limits; a modest honorarium.

____ 5. *Accountable communication*—open issues and conflicts between people are addressed early and fearlessly.

____ 6. *A management committee (eg, the MP, administrator, site managers, CFO, department heads)*—meeting every 2 weeks using accountability documents allowing each committee member and the board to see the status of all open projects.

____ 7. *Other meetings*—with appropriate frequency, duration, and content
- All hands (monthly to annual depending on scale)
- Departments (monthly)
- Providers (monthly)
- Committees/task forces (as needed)

____ 8. *An "action grid" or similar project accountability tool*—showing item, owner, deadline, and dated progress notes; updated bi-weekly and used as the core agenda for the management committee.

____ 9. *Written operational guidelines for all practice areas*—these standard operating procedures (SOPs) are updated regularly and memorialize the "one, agreed, best" way to do everything in the practice—force service consistency, formalize training, and advance the continuous quality improvement mission.

____ 10. *Quality assurance/performance improvement*—a standing committee that examines outcomes, utilization, facilities, and the customer experience, and focuses its attention on a current scope of work.

____ 11. *Root cause analysis*—the managers and board do not just look at surface symptoms but look for the "problem behind the problem" to revise the root causes of performance gaps.

____ 12. *Profit margin sufficiency*—practices with higher percentile profit margins (eg, above 40%) have the resources to seize opportunities, react to challenges, and weather fee cuts.

____ 13. *Income vigilance*—continuous, formal scanning for missed opportunities to reduce or share costs, boost incremental revenue, and add new ancillary services.

____ 14. *Capital access*—keeping no less than 3 months of cash and equivalents (eg, lines of credit, personal funds) at the ready as a business "shock absorber" for third-party payment delays, transient doctor disabilities, etc.

____ 15. *Risk management vigilance*—scanning the environment for potential threats and lining up mitigation resources before they are needed (eg, compliance audits, insurance products).

____ 16. *Financial and volumetric data analysis*—both traditional financial statements and PM system reports, plus derivative graphical aids, are used to spot adverse trends early.

____ 17. *Benchmarks*—pushed down the chain of command, memorized, and tracked at appropriate intervals. Positive values are used to reassure the board about the company's favorable performance; any adverse values are a trigger for timely response.

_____ 18. *Revenue cycle management*—ensuring that we are getting paid fully and in a timely manner for the work we do, and billing department work is done competently and efficiently.

_____ 19. *Sufficient practice facilities*—ensuring practice development is not choked off by a lack of space, equipment, or technology.

_____ 20. *Mid-level manager development*—ongoing, effective efforts with sufficient formality and time commitment to help department managers, at every career stage, advance their skills.

_____ 21. *A marketing mindset*—with staff at all levels, conscious of the desired growth rate and the practice's mission to preserve or increase its market share—includes a continuous focus on customer service, continuity of care, referral outreach, and an appropriate array of direct-to-consumer efforts.

_____ 22. *A career coaching mentality*—an approach in managing both providers and support staff cohorts that focuses on individual development.

_____ 23. *The use of external expertise*—drawing on outside subject matter experts (eg, peer practices, professional advisors, readings, continuing education meetings) to find and solve problems and to stay current.

_____ 24. *Passive income development*—through the development of ambulatory surgery centers, opticals, employee providers, etc.

_____ 25. *Intentionality*—rather than drifting from one random expedient to the next, the practice intentionally pursues a logical, linear progression of opportunities.

• • •

When you have finished, go back and add up your score. The maximum score is 100 points. Use the overall score, as well as your lowest per-item scores, as the jumping-off point for an internal discussion about needed improvements.

CHAPTER 2

The Big Picture

Imagination was given to man to
compensate him for what he is not;
a sense of humor to console him for what he is.
—Sir Francis Bacon

Of the Five Domains of Practice and Life

You've probably been asked a few thousand times by well-intentioned parents or competitive siblings, "So, how's it going? What are your plans for the future?" Chances are, even now, you answer these questions by rote—and a bit defensively—just as you have since you were a college sophomore. "Oh, I don't know. It was a pretty good year. If I can have another one like it next year I'll be happy. Beyond that, we'll see."

That is a perfectly acceptable white lie to tell your relatives, but a complete disservice to your professional and business life if you're a practice owner. Even if you

Pinto JB. *Simple: The Inner Game of Ophthalmic Practice Success, Second Edition* (pp 5-23).

run the smallest practice in town, success obliges that you look yourself in the mirror at least annually and get real about the future.

Where to start? This business and personal self-examination is something you can divide and conquer.

There are five logical domains, which I discuss in the following section. Each of these flows from one to the other. You can't effectively decide on strategic or tactical goals for your practice until you have clarified your personal and financial goals—or until you and any fellow surgeons in your practice have developed a sufficiently intimate relationship to be able to align your interests as partners.

• • •

Personal Goals

Take a deep breath. This is the hardest question: What do you want to see, have, do, be, experience, and give away in your remaining sentient, physically active years?

The average ophthalmologist is now a male in his 50s. Imagine that's you today. Here's the countdown: You will practice for about another decade—and transit about 50,000 remaining patient visits. You have perhaps 20 or 30—or if you're *very* lucky 40—years left to walk without a cane, hear without an aid, or speak without having someone younger remind you what you were talking about.

You have already worked out how to earn a living and live within it. But if your life is not yet meaningful—and many surgeons in their 50s tell me they are not yet living meaningful lives—how will you make it so? You have already used up more years than still remain.

How is your work–life balance? When will you retire? More importantly, to what will you retire? What are the values that help you prioritize how you will spend the fast-ebbing balance of your life?

When I visit with clients, these personal questions are often much more difficult to answer than those related to the science or business affairs of medicine. And yet, these are the questions that must be answered before you can frame up and intentionally pursue a coherent professional life.

Personal Financial Goals

In the context of your personal goals, which may be major or modest, are you on track with earnings? Are your earnings and savings aligned with your lifestyle costs before and after retirement? If these are not yet aligned (and chances are, you need more income to reach your personal goals—this is America, after all, where needs are often endless), there should be a feedback loop to the practice's strategic and tactical dimensions, which will allow greater active or passive earnings.

Once you are clear about your personal goals, the associated financial details can be reduced to very plain, A-B-C terms. You or someone you know may have a situation like this:

- Dr. Smith is 55; she wants to retire at 65.
- Smith was a bit late in making financial plans, and it appears that in 10 years she will be $500,000 short of the funds she needs to retire.
- After accounting for a modest appreciation of her current and future savings, Smith's CPA determines that she needs to earn (and save) an extra $400,000 over the next decade.
- Smith needs to earn an extra $40,000 every year for 10 years.
- Since most practice costs are fixed, there is only a 40% variable overhead load on every incremental dollar she brings into the practice. So, to clear $40,000 a year, she needs to generate about $67,000 in extra collections.
- She collects an average of $160 in net revenue per patient visit.
- At $160 per patient visit, that comes to 419 extra visits for the year. After accounting for vacations and meetings, Dr. Smith only needs to transit an extra nine patients per week to meet her goals.

Transpersonal Goals

Unless you are in solo practice, your personal and personal financial goals must be coordinated with, and then remain in sync with, those of your partners.

Here are some examples of how partners get out of sync with each other:

- By skipping meetings, and then complaining about board decisions
- By voting for your interests rather than the best interests of the practice
- By voting in the boardroom, and then undermining the board's final decision among support staff because it goes against the way you voted
- By taking excess personal time, after everyone has agreed that partners are limited to 6 weeks off each year
- By unreasonably writing off refraction and testing charges, pushing more overhead costs to your partners
- By pressuring your colleagues to purchase a nonessential new technology for your clinic, even when the practice's finances are tight
- By excessively competing with the newest doctor to join the group, even if 15 years ago the senior partner cannibalized their schedule to give you a leg up

Every practice's board is different. Some lucky surgeons sing "Kumbaya" and share rotating partner dinners at each other's homes. Many more, a majority, frame up practical working relationships that fall short of close social friendships, but that still allow for effective teamwork. Thankfully, very few despise and avoid their colleagues like bickering spouses. Such conflicts must be dampened—or the source of conflict removed—to be able to effectively operate a contemporary ophthalmic practice in these fast-shifting times.

Strategic Goals

"Strategy" and "tactics" are often confused and transposed. Simply said, strategic goals are couched more sweepingly and over longer time horizons, including the following:

- Where will we be in 5 to 10 years?
- What will our environment be like? Will we have access to patients and health insurance dollars?
- What will be our geographic span?
- What services will we add or subtract?
- What will the provider mix look like—ODs vs MDs/DOs?
- What will be our growth rate? (If revenue doesn't grow at least 4% per year, you will be losing market share.)
- Will we have firm institutional ties or remain neutral and "Swiss" in our market? Can we remain neutral or must we sell out to a larger player?
- How will we handle succession?

Only after the answers to these larger questions are clear can we address the more granular, tactical choices.

Tactical Goals

Tactics are actions, planned and performed over shorter time horizons in the service of your practice's strategic goals. In the previous example of Dr. Smith, who needs to transit nine more patients a week in order to meet her financial goals, the logical tactics would include:

- Inform the staff of her goals and get buy-in.
- Change the template to accommodate three more patients per clinic day.
- Change overtime policies to allow one tech to stay half an hour late as needed.
- After the new template has been running for a few weeks, pull the staff together and iron out any wrinkles, such as: Is the clinic running behind? Are patients complaining of too-little face-to-face time with the doctor? Is the billing department keeping up with a slight increase in workloads?

Tactics have to be triaged, just like medical care. You will not be able to do everything this year.

• • •

Striving is important, but be balanced in your striving. Goals are more about trajectory than target. Few of our greatest goals are fully realized, even by the most talented among us. The value and purpose of great goals, "push goals" as they're often called, is not to achieve them precisely, but to meander toward them approximately.

Attaching excessively to an outcome (ie, "I will live in a penthouse and drive a Ferrari by the time I'm 50") may keep you from enjoying the perfectly terrific consolation prize of driving a Lexus up the driveway of your comfortable suburban ranch house.

On your path, cleave to Hemingway's counsel, "It is good to have an end to journey toward; but it is the journey that matters, in the end."

Of Paying Attention

The Spanish philosopher José Ortega y Gasset said, "Tell me to what you pay attention and I will tell you who you are."

One summer I went hiking in the High Sierra, that north-south spine of mountains transecting California. The scenery was sublime. The trails were steep. And the air was quite thin. It was for that reason, around noon one day, that I stopped for lunch in a shady grove, sitting on the ground with my back against a comfortable boulder. Only about 15 feet from the trail. In plain sight.

My lunch was so relaxing that I had a nap for dessert.

I awoke a short while later, but remained very still for the next 2 hours. In that time, about 50 fellow hikers—some in groups, some alone—walked past me. Without one exception, each person droned on, feet plodding. Eyes focused on the ground ahead. Not one person looked my way or noticed I was there. They also didn't notice the two deer that grazed for 30 minutes on the far side of the trail. Or the family of jays, scratching nearby in the sand.

As a kind of "ophthalmic field naturalist" for the last many years, I can give the same report about most client offices. Far too many ophthalmologists and their management staff trudge along, overlooking the details of their environment. One foot in front of the other. Oblivious to much of what's going on in their practices.

This oversight is costly, both objectively in bottom-line business performance terms and subjectively in the medical quality deficits that are ignored and left to blemish patient care.

Assembled below, in no particular order or priority, are things you may be overlooking in your slog through each clinic day. This rundown is not meant to be a checklist, but a meditation. And a wake-up call. Do not race off and see if these things are present or absent in your practice—but rather, use these examples to punctuate any dissatisfaction you may have with your own attentiveness and to spur improvements at every level.

- How happy is your first-year associate with their posting in your practice? When they let out a sigh about their tech coverage, were they just venting or asking for a solution? Was their last 4-day weekend really a vacation, or were they interviewing in another practice? Is there something you could do this month to increase the odds that they will graduate to partnership … and contribute to the development momentum of your clinic?
- Are your incentives as a provider aligned with those of your staff? What reward do they get for improving their job skills or transiting more patients? How do they feel, 1 week after another pay freeze is announced, when you drive up with a new car? How does that feeling translate in the interaction they will have a few minutes from now with their work-up patient in Room 3?

- It's the end of another workday, all 500 or so minutes of it. Are you conscious of how much or little of each minute was engaged in income-producing or quality-improving activity? Have you stayed on the clinic floor and walked directly from patient to patient today, or wandered into your private office between most encounters? Has every patient needing a supplemental test been so-ordered? Has every patient received a definitive return-to-clinic order?
- Nearly half of all doctor and lay staff hires fail. Do you fail more or less often than others? Do you know why? Who in the practice is responsible for the success or failure in this critical area? What are their measurable, accountable goals?
- Just about anywhere you stand in a busy eye clinic, if you look and listen, you will observe numerous staff–patient interactions all taking place at the same time—a kind of customer service symphony. What's the overall tone? Purposeful ... friendly ... competent? Or chaotic ... grim ... bumbling? If we could give this symphony a score from 1 (wretched) to 10 (awesome), what would the score be today? What is our capability? Why aren't we there yet?
- During your next surgical consultation, try to step away from yourself and observe how you are interacting with the patient in your exam chair. What do you say? How do you say it? How do they react? How about the patient's accompanying family member? Might a subtle shift in body language, or a clearer, more affirming turn of phrase, mean the difference between a patient settling for standard care or choosing advanced surgery?
- As an eye surgeon, you've mastered at least one thing—surgery. So, you know what mastery feels like. How does ***that*** level of mastery compare with your understanding of and control over your clinic's business affairs? Are you a financial master yet? A project management master? A master at motivating personnel? You went to class to become an ophthalmic master—what classes are you taking to master your enterprise?
- Practices, from year to year, rarely stand still. Is your practice on the way up? Or is it on the descent because the founders are senescing—and not being replaced by young doctors of equivalent ambition and work ethic? Can this fall be arrested and reversed? Should it?

• • •

Your entire professional career will be composed of nothing but successes and lessons. How much attention you pay to the latter will expand the number of the former that you enjoy. Pay attention. It pays.

Of Career Management

What do you possess, really, when you leave formal training and enter the world as a newly minted ophthalmologist? Knowledge, to be sure—in abundance. A few scars. Enough wild-haired stories to fill a small novel, if you've been lucky and well rounded. But what you ***really*** possess is a brand-new, baby career.

In the 30 or more career years that stretch out ahead to the horizon, if you're at all ambitious, you'll likely serve more than 25,000 different patients. You will perform more than 150,000 examinations and more than 5000 major surgical cases—for which you'll be paid well in excess of $25 million, and get to keep, after expenses and taxes, perhaps $6 million or so. With any kind of discipline and care, you'll be able to retire, early if you like, with a net worth of several million dollars and the deep satisfaction that comes with doing your best and serving others well.

Or, if you do not manage your career especially well, if you passively float through your professional life, then you'll work less fruitfully, earn substantially less, and retire later and poorer than you might prefer.

The choice between these two divergent outcomes is ***entirely*** yours.

Active Career Management

"Doing" a career is not like "doing" cataract surgery. Unlike the plan you've been taught to craft stepwise for each of thousands of surgical cases, you've had no formal training and no logic tree to follow in navigating your career. And, of course, you only have one single career to get perfectly right the very first time you try. Thankfully, you have years and years to correct any errors you make along the way—and few mistakes are completely irreversible. Let's explore the biggest success and failure factors.

There was a time when every new ophthalmic grad had just a couple of offers of employment, from a couple of almost-equal contenders. Today, the number of offers per new grad has increased somewhat, while the diversity of opportunity has exploded: small and large single-specialty group practices, multispecialty practices, corporate centers, staff-model HMOs, teaching positions, and veterans hospitals and related governmental service. Most of the offers out there are solid enough, like the institutions behind them. But today there's a much higher percentage of career deathtraps than ever before, such as the following:

- Corporate centers too-thinly capitalized to make payroll, much less market your services
- Institutional positions in highly politicized departments, where you'll spend as much time dodging bullets as doing surgery
- Private practice opportunities, where you're promised the moon verbally, but end up with pixie dust, no partnership, and little wage equity—until you leave only to be replaced by the next naïve short-termer
- Well-meaning practices that hire a partner-track associate before they have enough business to support this next surgeon

Remember that you are not hiring on as some factory hand, with a union boss to protect you if you're mistreated. As a free-agent ophthalmologist, you are a union of one, and you need to think that way well before you sign off on your employment agreement. At the same time your prospective employer is vetting you, you should be vetting the employer. If you're being considered for a partner-track position, you should have access to at least some of the following due diligence information once you have been accepted as a finalist for the position:

- Financial statements for recent years
- Production and income statistics for each doctor over the past couple of years
- The provider-to-population statistics in the practice's service area
- A copy of any business or strategic plans extant
- A copy of a typical partner employment contract and compensation methodology
- A summary of prospective partnership terms
- A written description of efforts that will be undertaken to help you build a practice
- The names and contact information of any partner-track associates who have left the practice in the past 5 years

Not long ago, doctors signed employment agreements with a blind eye to the details of the contract or the strength of the employer. Increasingly, new grads and mid-career job candidates are spending thousands of dollars for help to comb through this due diligence data—cheap insurance given what's at stake.

• • •

Let's assume you've now taken a job—any job. What's the next stage of actively managing your career? It's simple, really. For real success, you need to work harder than you ever thought possible. You have to work and think like an owner, even if you aren't one yet.

Your first years as an ophthalmic associate are more profitable and less gruesome than the first years you would have spent as a junior associate in a law or accounting firm. All the same, it really helps to jump-start your practice by self-imposing a level of workaholism that very few surgeon-bosses would impose on you or themselves. By exceeding their expectations—and perhaps your own, as well—you'll jump-start success for the balance of your career. And this work should not be all clinical. In the first 5 years of your career you should be putting an extra 8+ hours a week into marketing, outreach, and learning the business of eye care.

Actively decide, all along the way, your desired balance between work and the rest of your life. Most young surgeons I know start out their careers affirming, "I'm not going to get into my father's rut—he worked 55 hours a week as a doctor … I'm not working over 40 hours." Check back in 10 years later, and this same doctor, rounding the corner to middle age and a maxi-mortgage, is probably treading their dad's same footsteps. So it goes.

In truth, working *smarter* will only go so far in today's medical business climate. In a fixed cost business, it is simply too punishing financially not to work more than 40 hours per week in most settings. Fortunately, what takes hold of almost every ophthalmologist by this stage in life is a kind of "work hardening" that allows you to see a few more patients every year but not feel any more exhausted, because you're becoming more efficient and tougher—both physically and mentally.

Although at 45 you may have 20 or more work years still to go, decide as early as possible when you want to retire, even if it's a provisional goal. Get professional help, in the form of a fee-only financial planner or accountant, to determine the annual savings rate you need to hit this goal. Along the way, and especially during your high-earning/high-spending years, be sure to manage your lifestyle costs. You should be arranging your affairs to live on less than 80% of your net after tax income, investing the rest for retirement and a rainy day. If your income fluctuates wildly (as in the typical elective or snowbird practice), do not delude yourself and craft a lifestyle indexed to your best years—be extra conservative.

Are you as efficient as you could be? Once you feel you've mastered everything in gross survival terms, and you're making a satisfactory living, it may be time to fine-tune your practice. Regularly examine how you're spending your time, from two perspectives. First, what is your ***net income per hour?*** In the typical setting, this figure is in the range of $150 to $500, once you figure in administrative time. Second, look at things existentially. What is your ***net enjoyment and satisfaction per hour?***

Career management success can be measured by seeing the profit you generate per hour going up, along with the progressive delegation of those tasks you find least pleasant or least suited to your skills and demeanor.

The ophthalmologists I know who are happiest in their careers are those who are flexible. They do not get inappropriately angry with minor staff errors, confused patients, work-ins, or cancellations. They exert control where they can: voting on the practice board, going off to get subspecialty training, or learning about the nuances of the business. They do not get bent out of shape by things beyond their control, like Medicare fee reductions or the addition of another competing doctor to the community. They enjoy teamwork in all its forms and can shift happily from leadership to "followership."

Doctors in nominal control of their career write down their goals and review their lists often. These goals, to be most useful, are measurable and objective. Not, "I will do more surgery," but "By this time next year I will average 25 cataract cases per month."

Doctors who craft great careers are often wide-ranging in their interests. They're as drawn to reading a book on business, history, or art as they are to reading the technical manual of their latest diagnostic equipment. They can relate to a wide range of staff, patients, and fellow providers.

And, lest you think that success is either an always "on" or "off" switch, some of the doctors I know today who are the most successful in global terms have not always enjoyed such success—they rose from failure. Like the client of mine who was abused in a group practice setting, but who went on to spectacular success in solo practice. Or the doctor who went down miserably with a failing management company, but rose right back up again from this disaster.

We are all paid for value, or at least the perception of value. Most subspecialists are more valuable than most generalists. But even if you missed out on subspecialty training, it doesn't necessarily mean you have to forego subspecialty-level success. Make a list of what you currently do for patients, and a second list of what you refer out. Do you need fellowship training to competently perform your own panretinal photocoagulation laser or cosmetic lid surgery? Perhaps not. Increase your skill set, increase your value to the patient, and your career potential will rise.

It vastly helps your career (if not your sense of well-being) for you to fake yourself out a bit and start each day with a healthy dose of fear: "I'd better get going here, or … our profits are going to falter … our competition is going to climb right up our backs … my skills are going to get rusty." This especially helps you fight the complacency that comes with mid-career success. If you haven't yet developed the next big goal to drive to in your career, at least keep the engines roaring to stay ahead of the pack behind you.

• • •

Average ophthalmologists—perhaps like the average person—do not think very often or very deeply about their motivations to continue in practice or how well they're progressing in their work. Thoughtful ophthalmologists think often about their progress. They figuratively hover above themselves in the course of a day, saying, "Nice catch," or "I guess you pretty much muffed that one … try harder next time." I've found that this internal, self-coaching dialogue is one of the common signposts of the most successful surgeons I know. They've replaced external drivers—professors and parents—with their own internal patter.

Thinking consciously about your career and managing it actively, you'll come to realize that to be happy with your career as an ophthalmologist, you need to love one or more of the four main dimensions of this kind of work:

1. The act of serving and helping each patient
2. The intellectual and tactile stimulation of the service you provide
3. The acclaim and social position that medicine brings you
4. The financial comforts and security that medicine can generate

Of course, which of these you love best is a measure of your development and evolution as a person, and your sense of security in the difficult reimbursement environment that lies ahead. To which of these motivations are you most attached?

The signs that you are not managing your career well are simple to spot:

- Your sense of career satisfaction rises and falls in lockstep with your monthly income.
- You dread coming into work each day and find every possible excuse to lighten your schedule.
- You wince more than once or twice a week when you have to enter a room to serve a difficult patient.
- At the end of the day, you are consistently happier that the day is over than you were in the morning when the day was starting.

Satisfaction is what's left over when you compare your reality to your expectations. Eye surgeons who enter medicine with low expectations, and who then perceive that they gain much, are the happiest and most satisfied in the profession.

• • •

I reference the following quote from poet Kahlil Gibran's *The Prophet* several times a year when I'm called by surgeons who have truly reached the end of their ropes, wondering if they should leave the profession altogether:

> Always you have been told that work is a curse and labor a misfortune … if you cannot work with love but only with distaste, it is better that you should leave your work and sit at the gate of the temple and take alms of those who work with joy.

How's your own "joy factor" doing? Do you love your work? Unfortunately, I think that even the happiest eye surgeons I know wake up each morning, more often than most professionals, asking the question, "What's next?" It's too bad, especially when you consider that many eye surgeons picked ophthalmology because it offered more than other specialties: more income, better lifestyle (less call duty), and almost universally favorable patient outcomes.

Take This Career Development Test

How satisfied are you with your career progress? For each of the five questions below, choose an answer that best fits you. Tally up your score, and derive an average A, B, C, D, or F letter grade—a "career GPA," if you will.

1. Compared to where I thought I would be *overall* at this point in my career I am:
   A. Significantly ahead of my expectations.
   B. Somewhat ahead of my expectations.
   C. About even with my expectations.
   D. Somewhat or significantly *behind* my expectations.
   F. An abject failure as an ophthalmologist.

2. I believe that those people who live in my *professional* world (eg, my patients, staff, colleagues, advisors) think I am:
   A. Among the most caring, accomplished, and exceptional doctors they have ever met.
   B. Easily within the top third of doctors they know.
   C. About average, as ophthalmologists go.
   D. Probably not the sharpest scalpel on the Mayo stand.
   F. A good candidate for retraining in a different, less-taxing profession.

3. I believe that those people who inhabit my *private/personal* world (eg, my friends, spouse, children, parents) think I am:
   A. Among the luckiest people in the world, who not only has a great job I relish and do well, but who also strikes a nice balance between my professional and personal lives.
   B. One of those fortunate people who gets to enjoy what I do for a living and does a pretty good job at it.
   C. Just like most people, with things I like and dislike about my job ... but not so frustrated that I'm about to rock the boat and change what I do for a living.
   D. Basically miserable about my career, something that spills into every other part of my life.
   F. On the verge of abandoning medicine.

4. It's a weekday morning. When I'm getting up and ready for work I usually feel (answer as a composite of your feelings about your surgical and clinical and management work):
   A. Alert, happy, and eager to get to the office/operating room.
   B. Perky, but with one or two fleeting thoughts of unpleasant tasks ahead in the day.
   C. Relatively cheerful, but aware that on many days there may be some things I'd really rather be doing instead of coming into work.
   D. Like dreading the day, gritting my teeth, and basically willing myself to go through the motions.
   F. Like calling out for the rest of the year or telling my staff I'm not coming in.

5. When I get to the end of my workday (or night!), I generally feel:
   A. Tremendously satisfied, as though there was almost nothing I could have done that day that would have been as fulfilling; I'm energized for whatever the rest of the day may hold.
   B. Satisfied and proud of a job well done, but eager to move on to what is a comparatively more pleasant part of my day.
   C. Terribly glad that the day is over and I can go home and recuperate.
   D. Completely spent, and already dreading the fact that in just a few hours another unpleasant day will be starting all over again.
   F. On the verge of collapsing at my desk.

Using the familiar grade point average, what was your overall score? Does it work out to a "B+"? A solid "A"? An "F"? Is it lower than you would like?

There are lots of other ways of keeping score in the career success race. Some ophthalmologists I know have gotten their greatest career tickle by developing a showcase facility. One Eastern doctor sinks more than 15% of every dollar he collects into his architectural award-winning masterpiece (4% to 6% is more typical). His net profit margin is only about 20%. Yet, he is so pleased with his decision to develop a showcase facility to work in every day that he's willing to cut back on other lifestyle costs.

Another doctor I know loves his practice team. His large staff contingent is among the brightest I've ever met as a group. And the most expensive—he spends about 45% of his cash flow on staff wages and benefits (under 30% is more typical). But he is tremendously fulfilled career-wise.

As they say, free time is the ultimate luxury. I know a bachelor doctor who takes a luxurious 20 weeks off each year. His practice performance shows it—his annual pretax income is well under six figures, yet he's probably one of the happier surgeons I've met in the last 23 years. He's almost never fatigued and has plenty of time for travel and other personal interests. Yet some would gauge him a failure at his career.

There are several other qualitative and existential career measurements—metrics that go beyond the raw numbers of dollars or patients or cases.

Some doctors who dislike the grind of routine clinical care (but relish surgery) hire medical ophthalmologists and optometrists. In practices with older patient populations (or patients derived from consumer advertising), these extenders are well-accepted as a surrogate for most visits with the surgeon, allowing them to do what they love best. So long as patients are satisfied and outcomes are high, the potentially lower overall percentile profit margins from this practice model are perfectly acceptable, especially since the net profit to the surgeon-owner of such practices can be higher, since their own time is used more productively.

For other doctors, the reputation of patients, staff, and peers is paramount. These are the doctors who invest their own time and money for outside help on quality assurance initiatives, staff education, and satisfaction studies. Of course, real progress in quality often begets commercial success. So, if a practice owner focuses on quality first, the bottom line tends to take care of itself.

Good partnering, though rare, results in some of the highest levels of surgeon satisfaction I witness around the country. To the extent it can be learned, and I believe it can, the elusive ability to find and cultivate superior partner relations should be on the curriculum of every medical school and residency program. Professional partnerships are at least as complex and prone to disharmony as marital partnerships. If you and your practice partner are killing career satisfaction for each other, it may be time for counseling or divorce, rather than years of continuing struggle. I end up spending a good portion of every client session on dispute resolution, which must precede any meaningful practice development work.

Of the Intentional Practice

I'm thinking about a client. He's in his 50s, pleasant and quite conforming with the status quo, probably going all the way back to the expectations and rules of his parents and first teachers.

He has absolutely no idea how he got where he is today. He simply put one foot in front of the other at the insistence of others, with little self-planning, without internalized expectations, without self-intention. So, it's not surprising that now he's asking for yet another outside opinion on what he should do with his life and practice.

It doesn't matter if your intent is to maintain the status quo of a modest practice or shoot for great professional heights—being more internally intentional (and not simply directed by those around you) ups the odds of achieving what you want. It also lowers your chances of winding up like this gentleman, Dr. Puppet, who after all these years is still unclear about what he truly wants for his professional life.

Before even thinking about what you want in strict practice terms, it's helpful to know what you want for your life. Listen to your own heart (or brain or guts—whatever you deem to be your wisest organ system).

As Henry David Thoreau wrote, "The price of anything is the amount of life that is exchanged for it."

If you are a practicing ophthalmologist, you have chosen a profession that obliged you to trade about 4 prime years of your youth for perhaps a $200,000 annual earnings premium over what you would have earned as a family practitioner. You can either spend that roughly $4 million in net-after-tax lifetime earnings premium on more take home pay and material possessions (by working the usual 45 hours a week as an eye surgeon), or you can trade that earnings premium in for more free time.

If you choose to work half time as an ophthalmologist, you will earn about the same as you would have working full time as a family doctor. You will also gain about 32,000 hours of free time to fill with passions that may exceed your passion for medicine. As a young person before starting a family (or as an older surgeon with the kids grown and the retirement fund nicely topped up), it's absolutely your choice. Are your actions today aligned with your intentions?

This same choice over ***how many*** hours of your life you spend at your profession can be applied to ***how*** these professional hours are spent. And that choice, in turn, reveals many other forks in the road like the following:

- The choice of financial abundance or mere sufficiency (with the former generally obliging greater time, greater risk, or both)
- The choice of being a durable employee or being an owner
- The choice of private vs institutional practice (working for a hospital, clinic, or government branch—or a life in academics)
- The choice of being on the technical cutting edge or being more conservative
- The choice of comprehensive or subspecialty practice
- The choice of rural or urban practice

If you are now 40-something or 50-something and in the middle years of your career, ask yourself: "Did I take the right path? Is this where I'm supposed to be? If not, what would it cost to take a do-over a couple of forks ago in the road? Am I willing to pay that price?"

Pursuing an intentional professional practice is not just for new graduates. In a career as financially abundant as ophthalmology, you can pivot to a different context. Even if you are now relatively locked down in mid-career (and mid-mortgage and mid-parenting), there are daily decisions to make that are more mindful and intentional. With a little bravery, and a bit more self-liberation and self-actualizing, you can really break out of old habits by the following:

- Firing tiresome patients and staff
- Starting clinic at 10 AM if you are really not a morning person
- Referring out complicated cases you currently grit your teeth through out of a sense of ego or pride
- Driving the exotic sports car you can readily afford, instead of the beater sedan that you think sends the "proper message"
- Leaving the bespoke suits, snug Italian shoes, and choking ties in the closet, and seeing patients in scrubs and Crocs

I know surgeons who, after considering their lives and becoming more intentional, are ramping up their businesses to mitigate falling profits. And I know several ophthalmologists—at every career stage—who are leaving for a life of mission work, for early retirement, or at least leaving for extended sabbaticals. Such self-actuated surgeons are among the happiest in America today.

It is important to surround yourself with people who will help you self-actuate. Is your spouse really just a substitute for a controlling parent, or someone who encourages your authentic growth? Do your practice partners encourage professional exploration or conformity?

Practice administrators can be cleaved into roughly two cohorts: those who want to build the practice of ***their*** dreams, and those who want to build the practice of ***your*** dreams. Pick the latter kind. Do not let a business manager with more ambition than you harass you into creating a professional life not suited to your temperament.

Finally, realize that the business counterpart of creating a more intentional personal and professional life involves writing a longer-term business plan. Indeed, the absence of formal business planning in many practice settings is simply a marker for a lack of personal life planning on the part of practice owners who are just drifting through life. The two domains are hinged to each other.

If you are stuck on what you want to do with your practice as a business, it can indicate a need to think more deeply about your life. And vice versa.

Of Practice Culture

Practices are like very, very small nations. Each has its own culture and truths, special words with special meanings, higher or lower standards, and greater or lesser levels of aggression in the pursuit of the practice's interests and goals.

Dictionaries dryly report that a "culture" is a set of ideas, beliefs, and ways of behaving of a particular group of people. But that doesn't quite cover it … not by half. Culture is juice. Culture is power. A purposeful, accomplishing culture, in a corporate context like an ambitious medical practice, possesses nothing less than a kind of group libido.

Personality drives behavior. Collective behaviors drive the practice culture. And practice culture drives everything else, including:

- How do we interact with patients and each other?
- What standards do we set for patient care and business performance?
- How do we respond when problems arise?

It's a core duty of practice leadership—whether you're the administrator, the MP, or a mid-level supervisor—to be sensitive to how your own personality and behavior resonates though the organization to frame up its composite culture.

If, as the administrator or lead doctor in your practice, you are ready to get out of the trenches and think at higher levels about the company you are crafting, there is no better place to start than an examination of culture. And the easiest way to begin is by asking questions about the various dimensions of your company's traits and conduct.

I've briefly unpacked 10 ophthalmic cultural dimensions in the following list. Read through these. Edit them. Add dimensions that are important to you and your board. Then use the resulting list as a jumping-off point for an internal discussion among practice leaders of the kind of culture you have today—and the kind of culture you would like to foster.

1. The ophthalmic mind has a notoriously short attention span. How far out is "the future" for you and your practice? Is your planning horizon the next few months, or do you plan with the next 10 years in mind? If your board snores when long-term strategic planning is on the agenda, do you acquiesce and move on to near-term projects, or does your board encourage you to help it think big thoughts?
2. How collaborative are you? Are decisions made at the top, or is decision making widely distributed? When the appointment schedule needs to be revised, do you make changes unilaterally or bring together selected staff and the affected provider and apply group-think to the best changes?
3. How do you set and measure the performance bar? Do you take what comes, or set specific growth and income goals? Do you have a tendency to set low, easy goals so that nobody is disappointed, or stretch and take some risk with some push goals, using these to draw your company forward to the next level of performance? Is practice performance gauged by industry benchmarks and a formal budget, or do you only examine performance at the year-end meeting?
4. How tidy are you? What are your physical plant standards? Are office facilities kept up to the level of a five-star hotel or a college dorm? Does someone patrol the parking lot for trash, and the reception area and restrooms for spills and disorder? Do you hold your cleaning service to high standards or do dust bunnies and scuffs go untouched for months?
5. How accountable are people in your practice? Do doctors follow through on their promises? Are they disciplined with their paperwork and faithful with meeting attendance? Is everyone's "to-do" list in their heads, or are everyone's action commitments written down, each with a deadline?
6. How great a steward of resources are you? Is your mindset to be highly resource sparing, even parsimonious—even if it means you end up underinvesting, deferring needed maintenance, and starving great opportunities? Or do you spend a bit too freely, remembering a bygone era in eye care when profits were abundant, and overlooking the pivot that the wisest administrators have made to attend more closely to their duties as comptroller?
7. How standards-setting or permissive is your practice? When staff err, do you look the other way or take immediate (but proportionate and kind) corrective action? Does your practice operate "by the book?" Are protocols in everyone's heads, or do you write protocols down and stick with them? Does every doctor in your practice see patients as they please, or rather follow agreed care pathways?
8. Is yours a "learning organization?" Are you a student of how different people learn differently, and how sometimes it's best to invest extra efforts in a slow learner who will eventually catch on and *then* do things exactly as taught (instead of free-lancing and making you crazy the way some fast-learning, super-smart people

can)? Do people learn by shadowing others and asking questions, or do you have a formal, written syllabus and a step-by-step process for transferring knowledge?

9. Is yours a "ME" or a "WE" practice? Do you only admit "givers" as new partners, or do you have some "takers" on the board? Is your practice just a collection of soloists who tolerate being in a group so they can share a few expenses? Or—even if the average ophthalmologist is naturally singular—do you work to foster a cohesive team? What does your compensation methodology say about the share-and-share-alike culture of your practice?
10. Do you place a high priority on communication and back it up tangibly with lots of resources? Are meetings rare, or is much time invested in such gatherings (even at the cost of productive clinic time)? Have you transitioned from an oral to a written culture, with memos and minutes and organization charts and all the rest so that everyone is, quite literally, on the same page?

• • •

Your practice culture is unique and complex, a thick soup of changing ingredients, completely unto itself. And like soup, it can be spoiled or redeemed with a single change of ingredients. A technophobic physician who has been holding your practice back from electronic health records can return from one class at a national meeting with an epiphany, an apology, and a vote for progress. The addition of one pot-stirring staff member can make your practice's culture toxic in short order. The loss of a senior practice founder's leadership can send a once-fabulous practice into oblivion.

Of Vanquishing Chicken Little

The sky is falling, the sky is falling!
—Chicken Little

CLFS—*Chicken Little fatigue syndrome*—is on the march through the land of eye care.

If you are the typical administrator or MP today, you've spent the last few years getting good and lathered up, perhaps by now numbed up, from the nation's enduring economic woes and ever-pending Medicare fee reform. And that was before the pandemic hit in 2020.

Like many, you may be saying, "We're still here and doing well enough … maybe things won't change after all. Maybe we should stop worrying." If you're letting down your defenses, if you are less alert and less prepared, then you, too, may be developing CLFS.

As this book goes to press, economists are examining the intersect of the pandemic's hit to the economy and a US recession that was already looming. The most dour analysts—or are they the most prescient?—are renaming the "Great Recession of 2008," and all of the years since, the start of the "Great Contraction."

This camp believes that the national economy is not going to rebound post-COVID-19 in the usual fashion, back to 3+% growth rates. Rather than an accustomed next upward leg of the business cycle in the 2020s and beyond, some believe the economy is shouldering off and settling into a new and lower baseline.

A sustained lower economic baseline would compound every issue managers and practice owners have been nervously skirting for the last few years, such as:

- Annual deficits and total national debt would become a larger percentage of the gross domestic product (GDP), forcing budget cuts and putting entitlements like Medicare squarely in the cross-hairs.
- Unemployment would remain stubbornly high and middle class wages stubbornly low, curtailing optical and elective care purchases and reducing the rolls of the insured.
- Most alarmingly for those in eye care, health care costs would rise even further as a percentage of GDP (we are at about 19% now, half again higher than the rest of the industrial West), providing the political cover needed to float major reforms.

Even without ever-looming fee cuts, we're seeing cracks in the wall. In some markets, I have seen eye care providers offering all new patients a free eye exam. Staff hours are being shed. Capital purchases are being delayed. And staff wages have certainly been stagnant, even reduced in some settings, over the last decade.

If the economic Chicken Littles are more than a little bit right, it's time for you to shake off the torpor of CLFS and consider what you would do as a leader if things got truly ugly. If the fee cuts came in earnest. If, as in California during an earlier recession, the federal government sent you vouchers instead of bankable checks.

It's an interesting exercise to undertake for two reasons. First, you'll prove to yourself that we are nowhere near exhausting the possible mitigation strategies available in the event of severe entitlements reform. Second, you may even unearth a few tactics you can roll out today, even if Chicken Little turns out to be wrong.

Here, then is a starter list of what you and your practice could do if the sky truly fell. Some of what follows is pretty radical. This is not a list of recommendations, so much as an inventory of "life raft" options you could unpack in tough times.

- Double-up office facilities and staff. Many ophthalmologists practice with more square footage and staff than is absolutely necessary. Two can't work as cheaply as one, but two independent surgeons, each with 70% cost margins, can join forces to create a practice with 60% or lower cost margins.
- Expand hours and add part-time optometric providers. Most practices are open about 40 hours a week. Some as little as 30 hours. In contrast, general retailers are open 50+ hours per week. As an ophthalmologist you can do the same thing, without working any harder personally, by adding part-time optometrists in the evenings and weekends.
- Refocus on senior eye care. Seniors control an outsized percentage of personal net worth in America, and coincidentally harbor the most ophthalmic pathology.
- Broaden your skill set and service mix. If you have a flagging practice and refer out retinal, glaucoma, and plastics, retain at least some of these patients after polishing up any subspecialty skills which may have gone stale.
- Pull up roots and move to an underserved or more prosperous part of the country … or the world. There are a staggering 14 billion human eyeballs on the planet, and an enduring market demand to see clearly and not go blind. And even if you're reluctant to go offshore, there are still materially underserved markets in America.

- Start bartering. Ophthalmologists with skills in universal demand are in a much better position to trade than, let's say, an investment banker. A few eye surgeons I know already work some of their time in the casual economy. If your great grandfather was a doctor, chances are he swapped his share of medical care for chickens and pigs.
- Or, how's this for the ultimate in radical practice management? Drop out of the game almost entirely. Stop accepting all third-party payments. Reduce your fees to levels your patients can personally afford. At the end of each exam, hand the test results and chart notes to your patient and ask them to bring them back the next time they visits you or another doctor ... saving you the cost of records storage and retrieval entirely. Transfer your assets to your spouse and cancel your malpractice insurance policy ... have all patients sign off an acknowledgment that their doctor goes bare. Toss out the appointment template and shift to a purely drop-in clinic. (How's that for a paperless office?) You would have a practice that looks a lot like modest medical clinics in the rest of the world, and not just the underdeveloped world. I once visited a practice just like this in Paris that was humming along fine.
- At the same time that you're pulling radical business solutions out of the cabinet, reset your expectations. Very few administrators or surgeons I know expected to earn what they do today when they were back in college. For most of us, some of the happiest days of our lives were in college or graduate school, where we earned a few thousand dollars a year, ate way too many PBJ sandwiches, nursed sputtering clunkers down the road, slept on mattresses on the floor, and stacked up boards and cinderblocks to hold our stuff. Keep reminding yourself, "It will be alright."

CHAPTER 3

Leadership

Great boldness is seldom without some absurdity.
—Sir Francis Bacon

Of Simple Leadership

Leading is simple at its root, but rarely encountered in ophthalmology. As Ralph Waldo Emerson said, "Our chief want is someone who will inspire us to be what we know we could be."

Imagine a small, green visitor from Alpha Centauri (our closest solar neighbor) lands its space capsule in your practice parking lot next week. It shuffles along the sidewalk, opens your front door with effort, finds its way to your receptionist, Molly, and using the familiar interplanetary lingo, says, "Take me to your leader."

Does Molly know where to escort it?

Pinto JB. *Simple: The Inner Game of Ophthalmic Practice Success, Second Edition* (pp 25-42).

If you're the surgeon-owner or the practice administrator, and things are going according to plan, Molly should be heading directly to your office. You're the leader, of course. But are you?

Perhaps not.

If you hire and fire and sign the pay checks, this is sufficient to be someone's "boss," but not their leader. And you are not a leader if you merely look over workers' shoulders, chastise them for errors, or give them a new task to accomplish. You may be supervising or overseeing or managing, but you are not leading.

Mere "management" is not necessarily leadership. Leadership takes management to the next level. All effective leaders are excellent managers. Only a few managers are excellent leaders.

Bridging the gap between managing and leading is a very rare thing for MPs and administrative managers to accomplish. Becoming a leader is less an accident of birth (as many assume), and more a matter of study and emulation of great leadership by others, combined with personal trial and error.

"Natural" leadership is a myth. Being a great leader is most often an ***unnatural*** act, obliging that you reach beyond your narrow personal interests. Meaning, to sacrifice, when it's natural to take; to be a workaholic, when it's natural to be lazy; to be self-deprecating, when it's natural to puff yourself up.

Here is a very basic list, 10 hallmarks of leadership in an ophthalmic context. I didn't invent these concepts—your colleagues did—I merely wrote them down after many decades of observing the best leaders I've met in the business.

1. Being an effective MD-leader takes raw time—at least 8 added hours per week on top of your core job as an ophthalmologist. Time for communication and meetings, along with self-education and reflection about what works and what doesn't in your hands and in your unique setting. Effective administrators must be equally workaholic; 45 to 60 hours a week is not uncommon. As retired surgeon and industry icon Dr. John Corboy was fond of saying, "If you're not smarter than them other guys, you had better work harder and longer than they do if you want to get ahead."
2. If you want to be both a great manager and great leader, you do not have to think like General Patton or President Lincoln. Instead, think like a doctor. Gather information about a problem, make a decision, act on your decision, and revise tactics as indicated by how well the problem resolves.
3. Ophthalmic microsurgery is the domain of slow, cautious, 100% perfection. Ophthalmic leadership is the domain of well-intended, timely approximations of 80% perfect. Or less. Nobody dies or goes blind in the world of business. Be bolder and faster than you are natively comfortable with. Get on with it.
4. Tough-plus-fair wins the day. People respond best, and do their best work, for those leaders (eg, parents, teachers, bosses, politicians) who are inordinately tough but simultaneously fair. Think back to your own favorite leader—who, chances are, was not loose and easy in setting standards for you. You may have hated your parent or teacher at the time, but in hindsight you can see they were right and acting ultimately in your best interest.

5. As an ***ophthalmologist providing patient care,*** you are in a popularity contest and want 100% of patients and referral sources to love you. As an ***ophthalmic business leader,*** you are decidedly not in a popularity contest. And this is not a democracy, except among equal partners in a boardroom setting. Leading the practice is doing the right thing for the company, even if it makes you a bit unpopular.
6. Practice staff, like kids (although we do not want to overstretch the analogy), do best with binary leadership—a highly engaged MD leader and an equally engaged administrator—like unified, collaborating parents, a force to be reckoned with. This is true at all practice scales, from modest solo practices (ie, with one doc and one beleaguered office manager, or OM) on up to the largest private clinics in America (ie, with one medical director or MP and one senior-level CEO-director.)
7. The typical ophthalmology practice (unlike larger corporate environments where you would come up the ranks and serve under many mentors) does not provide a very effective setting for learning leadership. Backfill this gap by studying other industries. Read widely, especially the biographies of leaders in other spheres.
8. Effective leadership is at least as much about one's desire to lead, as it is about one's innate skill set. Do not elevate a junior staff member to a supervisory position—or a board member to MP—unless they really ***want*** the job. You have probably run into this problem already. Most practices have at least one mid-level manager (most commonly a head tech or head of billing) who is technically excellent, but who does a terrible job leading other people.
9. Take your fiduciary responsibility to the practice seriously. Think *"practice first."* Make decisions based on what is best for the practice and the patients, not what is best for you personally. If it's best for you to open up extra clinic or OR days to accommodate patient demand, do so, even though your personal preference may be to enjoy the time off. If it's best for your partner to get their way this year with a new piece of testing equipment instead of you—because that's what is best for the practice—do not be a grump about it.
10. In the present spooky environment, with lower fees and higher costs, and personal taxes on the horizon, it takes a highly disciplined leader to not mutter out loud throughout the day about how the sky is falling. Robert Louis Stevenson said, "Keep your fears to yourself, but share your courage with others." While it's perfectly appropriate to discuss your fears with your partners and administrator, your mid-level managers and especially your in-the-trenches staff should be spared the doom and gloom. Find your courage, even in the present situation, and share it.

• • •

Business guru Peter Drucker wrote, "One does not 'manage' people. The task is to lead people. And the goal is to make productive the specific strengths and knowledge of every individual."

Of Decisiveness

Some years ago I went out for dinner with a new client in his home town. We arrived and sat down, exchanging the usual pleasantries. During our conversation, the menus arrived. The waiter directed our attention to a nearby chalkboard with the daily specials. Our conversation then came to a halt, and for the next 15 minutes the client combed through his menu, looking back and forth, laboring from page to page, and then up to the chalkboard. The waiter returned to our table several times to ask, "Would you like to order?" Only after another quarter-hour had passed was my client ready to order dinner and, even in the midst of ordering, he changed his mind several times.

Over the next 3 days of working together, I observed the same indecisive behavior in this surgeon's practice. This otherwise very intelligent man, I'll call him Dr. Vacillate, was entirely uncertain about the path his practice should take, who he should hire next, the new services he should offer, or the operational improvements he should make.

Although Dr. Vacillate was an extreme example of indecision, I've found that the medical precision and hard certainty required of every eye surgeon—an exactitude reinforced through years of rote training—can inhibit decision making on the business side of the practice. Such indecisiveness can transfer from doctor to doctor and from the boardroom to the managers and staff, creating a culture of indecision and procrastination.

This is clearly disabling and works against the business interests of your practice. Let's discuss some approaches to identifying and treating the problem.

Here are some signposts of indecision:

- You gather reams of information, and then gather some more. But you put off committing to a decision.
- You ask everyone's opinion—even those who really are not informed on the matter at hand.
- Even though you know a decision is time-sensitive, you fail to set a firm deadline.
- As a manager or provider, you fail to delegate appropriate decisions to others in the practice … or …
- … you delegate even the most important decisions to others, because you can't make a decision yourself.
- You make a decision in the morning, and then waffle throughout the rest of the day, going back and forth about whether your decision is correct.
- You announce to everyone what you think to be a final decision, and then reverse course when you hear the slightest protest from staff or colleagues.

If these examples are uncomfortably familiar, here are a few strategies for improvement.

First, turn your concept of your problem with decision making around, and look at it from another direction. Perhaps the goal should not be to somehow buck up, stiffen your spine, and become more decisive, but to *simply reduce the amount of time you spend being indecisive.*

Ask people you trust for feedback: "Do you think I'm procrastinating or being indecisive about starting up our first satellite office later this year?" It may be that your personality is not at all indecisive, but that on the issue at hand you are simply exercising normal levels of prudence.

Some managers and surgeons I know make their best decisions only after writing out all the pluses and minuses in two side-by-side columns. There's something about putting pen to paper (or fingers to keyboard) that draws out your best thinking. If you still can't make a decision, set the plus and minus list aside for a couple of days and return to it.

Be sure you are applying sufficient numeric objectivity to your decisions. Most business decisions can be reduced to a math problem. Should we buy or lease new office space? Will adding a fourth exam lane increase our profitability and reduce waiting time? Is it time to hire a partner-track associate? If you find it hard to think mathematically, engage your accountant or other advisor to crunch the numbers.

Expand your analytic and problem-solving abilities. As a surgeon, you spent years learning how to differentiate one disease from another. You are absolutely clear about the "key performance indicators" of the human visual apparatus. Are you equally savvy about the key performance indicators of your practice as a business entity? Think of business problems as a kind of "company disease." You need to know the right kind of "lab test" to apply to effectively diagnose and treat a business problem. And you need to know the normative benchmarks and reference standards for a healthy business.

Here's an example. Let's imagine that profit margins have fallen from 50% to 35% in your practice over the past 8 years. If yours is a general ophthalmology practice in an urban setting, the 35% figure may actually be a very acceptable profit margin—and the old 50% figure was an anomaly. However, if you have a retinal practice with the same fiscal performance, you would have reason to be concerned and quite reasonable in wanting to bring the 35% figure back up to 50% or higher. Analysis of the problem might include:

- *A review of individual doctor work hours.* High fixed costs increasingly oblige that doctors either work a full week and curtail vacation time, or job-share to make sure that practice facilities are 100% utilized.
- *A review of provider efficiency and work intensity.* Is each doctor seeing a sufficient number of patient visits per session?
- *A review of the surgical density and testing/treatment utilization rates.* Have profits slumped because we're not providing every patient with needed care?
- *An analysis of the revenue yield per average patient encounter.* Are we lower than others in our specialty?
- *A review of contracts.* Are we on every available panel and being paid per our contracts?
- *A scan of billing practices.* Are we doing the work, but not getting paid for it?
- *An examination of staffing, facility, and other costs.* Are we using resources efficiently?
- *A competitor review.* Why are other practices growing faster than we are?
- *A marketing audit.* Are we as visible in our community as we need to be?

Unfortunately, for these and other problem-solving chores, even the best formal business education provides little more than a starting point for accumulating experiences that will help you make better decisions. If you're still at an early stage of your career as a lay manager, practice owner, or MP, you can accelerate the learning curve by reading widely in the vast, often case-focused business literature. By learning from the mistakes and successes of others, you'll be able to make better and faster decisions.

Ask often: "Do I have enough information to make a decision?" Management is the process of gathering information, making decisions, and then implementing. The quality of your decisions, the confidence you have in them, and the conviction with which you implement will all be improved if the underlying facts and figures you gather are sound.

Decisiveness is a matter of degree. Your decision-making tempo lies on a continuum between too slow and too fast, with "just right" somewhere in between. Making decisions with too much hesitation may frustrate both you and your team. But, ultimately, rushing to decisions can be far more disastrous to your practice than being a bit inconclusive at times.

• • •

Decision making in ophthalmology can be reduced to a simple, four-step process, as follows:

1. Have we gathered enough information to make a correct decision?
2. Is the contemplated decision ethically, legally, and morally sound?
3. Is the contemplated decision more profitable than the alternatives?
4. If we are stuck between two equally worthy options, are we letting anxiety impede progress? (If so, flip and coin and let's get on with it.)

The German philosopher Friedrich Nietzsche might have added a fifth step: "Once the decision has been reached, close your ears even to the best counter-argument." Not bad advice for your next board meeting.

Of Prioritizing and Implementing

As an ophthalmologist, by the time your formal training is completed, and after accounting for vacation time, you only have about 8000 work days left to accomplish your professional mission. In these 8000 days you have to build a staff team, construct a business enterprise, refine your mastery of a complex body of clinical knowledge, and use this mastery to serve perhaps tens of thousands of different patients, and twice as many eyes. That's it ... just 8000 days.

This time passes swiftly. If you're mid-career, you only have about 4000 work days left. In another decade, you'll only have perhaps 3000 work days remaining. And by the time you finish this book section you'll have used up another 5% or so of ***one*** of those precious days.

So, what can you do to extract the most value from each of these fleeting days? The first answer is to prioritize. And this prioritization flows downhill, from profound life goals to unremarkable practice minutia:

Life goals (eg, buy a mountain vacation home to retire in one day)

↘

Practice goals (eg, increase income by $35,000 per year)

↘

Practice projects (eg, get more optometrist referrals)

↘

Practice tasks (eg, call Dr. Edwards for lunch)

If you keep your eyes open to opportunity, hundreds of alluring new ideas arise every year—you only have time in your life to pursue a fraction of these ideas seriously. How do you know which opportunities are important? You have to know your long-term goals, which provide a critical context for focusing the limited hours of your day, and the limited days of your working life.

Consider the following scenario. Imagine you're a 48-year-old general ophthalmologist, who dreams of owning a five-partner, mixed subspecialty practice. You want to be the MP of this group, and then work hard in this role for 20 years if your health can hold out. You want to continue performing cataract surgery and pass along to your colleagues just about everything else. These goals are consistent with the following actions:

- Going to a national meeting and sitting in on courses related to being the MP of a group practice
- Directing your administrator to strengthen their financial training to be ready for managing a larger organization
- Getting good at delegating to middle management staff in the practice
- Calling a recruiting firm to cast a net for your first partner-track associate
- Hiring a personal trainer to increase your energy levels

These goals, to own a larger group practice, would ***not*** be consistent with the following actions:

- Going to a national meeting and taking courses related to medical retinal care. You'll be delegating such cases in the future, remember?
- Directing your administrator to learn now to scrub into surgery as a backup for your lead scrub tech. Such work would be a distraction from running a business for you.

- Holding on to lots of detailed projects instead of delegating. You're going to be too time-poor to do everything well by yourself.
- Failing to follow a diet and exercise regimen that will keep you vigorous well into your 70s.

Here's a practical pop self-test: Have your actions this past week, day-by-day, been consistent with the outcomes you desire? If not, you'll want to align these to the greatest possible extent. Before reading further, fill out this simple grid.

Actions I Have Taken in the Past Week	The Larger Goal I Hope to Accomplish Through This Action
I visited an old friend from my residency (who performs cataract surgery faster than I do) to learn how I can shift from two cases per hour to three or four cases, to make it financially viable to develop a modest ambulatory surgery center (ASC).	I would like to have my own surgery center one day and can't afford this unless I'm a more efficient surgeon.

Were the activities you wrote down in the left column aligned with the goals you wrote down in the right column? If not, what does this tell you about the way you're prioritizing your time? Do you need to adjust your goals (perhaps defining them formally for the first time in years), or better direct your actions to match your goals?

Sometimes the focus of your time and attention is not driven by your desires alone, but is bounded by practical realities. Let's say you would indeed love to develop an ASC. You've bought every book on the subject and go to every possible ASC course. You have hired a few consultants to review the prospects and get the same answer back each time: "You can't develop an ASC because (1) your case volumes are too low to support such a center, (2) your market is so small that you'll never build sufficient case volumes, and (3) the regulations in this state prohibit the development of private ASCs." In light of these facts, it would be foolish for you to keep attending ASC courses, reading ASC how-to guides, and hiring advisors. Adjust your dreams; find another kind of practical ancillary service (an optical perhaps, or an augmented diagnostic testing pod) and put your energies into these more achievable goals.

Managing Your To-Do List

You do not gulp down an entire steak dinner in one bite; instead, the meal is divided into discrete courses, and each mouthful is cut one bite at a time. Practice projects should be carved up the same way. Once you have prioritized the outcomes you desire, and have developed a list of projects, it helps to break each project down into its component parts.

A number of computer programs have emerged to automate your to-do list. Microsoft Project is a robust program designed for projects with hundreds of subroutines, as would be the case if you're a general contractor building a new office tower. Microsoft Outlook is a much simpler program, packaged with Microsoft Office, that allows you to arrange projects by initiation date, departmental area, or responsible party. But perhaps the simplest and most familiar approach is to use Word or Excel to create the following table.

Sample Action Grid

Action (Dated)	Who (One Person)	Deadline	Progress Notes (Dated)
October 2—Replace the worn carpet in the Akron main office	Susan	November 20	October 15—Carpet samples reviewed and order placed October 30—Installation scheduled for November 13 November 10—Date pushed back due to flood damage repair work

Here are a few simple rules to accompany the use of such a grid:

- Date all action items, which should be a complete thought—even someone from outside of the practice should understand what you have written down in simple, subject-predicate format.
- Each item should have a single owner, not a committee.
- The deadline should be a specific date in the calendar, not "spring."
- If an item is approved but tabled until later, enter the "tabled to ____" date in the deadline column.
- Make sure that all progress notes are entered and dated ***by each responsible party*** on a shared, open access drive at least 48 hours in advance of regular management meetings—then you can use the grid as both the agenda and minutes for such meetings.
- Highly confidential items should be moved to a separate grid.
- Completed items should be removed to a separate archive file and reviewed periodically by the practice's managers to ensure that completed projects continue to be closed.

• • •

Whatever system you use—from a worn-out legal pad, to a dedicated computer program—it's critical to foster an *accountable* environment, where all action item "owners" feel truly responsible for their line items and where there is a formal consequence for not carrying out an agreed task. By starting with a clear understanding of the desired long-term outcomes for your life and practice, you'll find yourself and your staff spending more time on purposeful activity and less time on busywork that robs each day of the precious hours you need to accomplish your dreams.

Of Teamwork

The *Cambridge English Dictionary* defines a *team* as "a number of people or animals who do something together as a group." That's close enough for our purposes here (and given the behavior of some staff and doctors, perhaps a little too close to the truth in some settings). The same source says that *teamwork* is "work done by several associates, with each doing a part but all subordinating personal prominence to the efficiency of the whole." We'll go with that, too.

Every practice agrees with the concept that taking a team approach is a core requirement for providing great patient care. Most administrators work very hard in a day-to-day task sense to foster teamwork. But very few practice teams call a time out in the game to agree on just what constitutes superior teamwork, and to nail down missing elements. Therefore, I've done that for you here, with this simple Teamwork Assessment.

This list of attributes of great teamwork is by no means complete, and no practice could be expected to have high scores in all of these areas.

Score each item on this 40-point list based on the following scale:

5 I strongly agree with this statement.
4 I agree with this statement.
3 I am neutral... I neither agree nor disagree with this statement.
2 I disagree with this statement.
1 I strongly disagree with this statement.

_____ 1. Everyone on our practice team understands the historical context of our organization and where we've come from.

_____ 2. We have a written plan so everyone knows where we are heading in the future; group goals are clear.

_____ 3. We understand the rules of the game and how to keep score. We play to win and celebrate our wins, both large and small.

_____ 4. We communicate well with each other, and we are especially good at listening.

_____ 5. We all understand the roles ("positions") that everyone plays on the team.

_____ 6. As "players" on the same team, we show respect and appreciation for each other, up and down the ranks.

_____ 7. Managers in our practice personally demonstrate good teamwork to the rest of the team.

_____ 8. The doctors personally demonstrate good teamwork to the rest of the team.

_____ 9. We have fun and enjoy playing "the game" together as a group.

_____ 10. We reward staff at every level for their ideas, performance, skills, motivation of others, flexibility, willingness to try and risk failure, sharing, small improvements, etc.

_____ 11. We set standards and expectations for teamwork that are appropriate—with especially high standards for senior lay staff and partner doctors.

_____ 12. We are constantly developing a better group understanding of what the customer wants—and making service improvements in this context.

_____ 13. We hold a common mission to serve and delight all the fans in the stands: patients and their family members, payers, referring docs, employees and their dependent family members, etc.

_____ 14. We organize enough social interaction among the lay staff and doctors to develop great relationships with each other.

_____ 15. We educate ***everyone*** on the basics of ***every*** job, not only so we'll be able to cross-cover job functions, but so that we can have greater empathy for our colleagues' work environment.

_____ 16. We have developed specific performance expectations and standards and hold each other to these; we have created an environment where we each feel accountable to the team.

_____ 17. We understand the minimum standards of customer service and work together to exceed these.

_____ 18. We have boosted our investment in information technology to improve communication and productivity, and to reduce the frustration that comes with using outdated tools.

_____ 19. All members of the team are open to the input and reciprocal coaching of their colleagues. Our doctors are open to receiving and following through on the coaching efforts of their managers. Our managers are open to receiving and following the coaching efforts of the doctors.

_____ 20. We have a "playbook" (eg, the written personnel manual, operations manual, care pathways).

_____ 21. We get the team "psyched up," and elevate every teammate's reasonable expectations and enthusiasm about winning.

_____ 22. To watch us in action for 30 minutes, you would think we look more like a synchronized group than a collection of individuals running off in different directions.

_____ 23. We maintain a tempo that everyone can reasonably maintain.

_____ 24. We seek a steady increase in both the individual and the combined talents of the team; we work hard to improve weak links and give them a fair chance to improve.

_____ 25. We deal with each other with empathy; we do not make fun of weak links in the team, but rather help them.

_____ 26. When weak links on the team cannot be improved, we are not hesitant to remove them.

_____ 27. We do not withhold difficult information or "triangulate" (ie, when Mike complains to Ann about Mary).

_____ 28. We support decisive leadership and insist that our leaders lead.

_____ 29. We foster effective and appropriate "followership," the ability of team members to rally around the leader and respect their position always, even if from time to time we harbor concerns about the individual leader involved.

_____ 30. We are time-sensitive and do not dawdle once a course of action has been ordered.

_____ 31. We sacrifice for, and compromise with, each other.

_____ 32. We remember there is no "I" in "TEAM" and that "TEAM" stands for "Together Everyone Achieves More."

_____ 33. We each take responsibility—others can count on us.

_____ 34. We balance authority with responsibility and give our managers the authority they need to carry out their duties.

_____ 35. We take in all viewpoints and do not discount even the most outlandish ideas.

_____ 36. We are energetic and have great stamina.

_____ 37. We make everyone on the team feel important.

_____ 38. We play carefully, to avoid harming ourselves, others, or the company.

_____ 39. When any of us has our feelings hurt, we work through it and still stay in the game; we do not withdraw or quit playing.

_____ 40. Everyone plays—nobody sits on the bench for very long.

Total Score:__________

Add up your score. With 40 different attributes, and with up to 5 points each, there's a maximum score of 200. There is no objective scale that compares you to others, but this summary score can be a valuable internal baseline of your teamwork and can help point out areas to improve. It might be interesting to repeat this scoring instrument again in a year to track your improvement.

• • •

As a final—ideally group—exercise, select two or three weak aspects of your practice's teamwork which are suggested by your responses to the questions above. For each of these weak areas, write down specific goals and tactics to achieve them. Here is an example of what you might write down.

> No one on our team except the administrator and our partner doctors understand how we're doing as a practice. These "insiders" get the financial and volume performance data, but everyone else on the team has to guess if it's been a good or poor quarter compared to last year. To improve this, we're going to prepare a quarterly "dashboard" for the practice, containing five key benchmarks for this year vs last. These benchmarks will be: total patient visits, total surgical cases, a lay staff efficiency ratio consisting of total payroll hours divided by total patient visits, a doctor efficiency ratio consisting of patient visits per clinic hour worked, and the percentile increase or decrease in our collections. We will share this dashboard with every member of our staff at our quarterly all-hands meetings. Whenever our quarterly scorecard shows progress, we'll think up some creative way to celebrate our improvement as a group.

Of Abandoning Failed Projects

General George Washington's army lost more battles than they won—and yet they prevailed in the Revolutionary War. In a syndicated column, a different George—columnist George Will—wrote that America won the war not so much because of decisive victories, but because of its superior retreats, such as the one after the British landed on Long Island with an army larger than the local population of New York City.

It's useful to think of your practice career, panoramically, in the same terms. By the time it's over, you will have had some 30 years of victories and defeats, advances and retreats. For those of you reading this who are older, you already know that your career has been shaped as much by the strategic retreats you've taken, as by the advances. Whether in battle or in business, there's no dishonor in withdrawing to fight another day.

Take the example of a West Coast client, who some years ago left his large group practice to hang out his own shingle. Trouble is, he had no preparation—and no real interest—in the details of running a practice, something that had always been done for him in his large group. Compounding this was the open checkbook he gave his first OM to find and equip an office. "Mary" rang up bank and equipment leasing liabilities—all of it with personal, not corporate, recourse—exceeding $1 million before the practice was 6 months old. It was a mountain of debt, and this surgeon spent the next 3 years trying to keep up with it. But they do not give out prizes for going broke slowly. In the end, the only reasonable course was for this gentleman to declare bankruptcy and accept a partner-track position with another large group. After a strategic retreat from an untenable position, he's happy and prosperous today ... and almost out of debt.

There are many such strategic retreats in modern practice. One of the most common today is the retreat that lower-volume refractive surgeons are making from cornea-based vision correction surgery. Hundreds of ophthalmologists who thought it would be both professionally interesting and highly profitable to add a modest LASIK service to their largely geriatric businesses are realizing that it's easier in most circumstances to grow by adding services of interest to your existing customer base than it is to find an entirely new pool of customers.

The same can be said—and a good deal more harshly—about the shopping basket of cosmetic and aesthetic services like dermabrasion, facial peels, and even elective cosmetic (as opposed to functional) blepharoplasty. These are services that seem intuitively sensible to add, right? But they end up being empirically wrong in almost every practice setting. With very few exceptions, the profitability of these services is terrible compared to mainstream ophthalmic care. As a result, most minor cosmetic procedures offered in ophthalmic practices are break-even at best, and at worst are an expensive gift to your staff and your spouse's social circle.

Remember that the acid test for adding a new product or service to your practice is: "Will this either measurably improve the quality of care we offer our patients or ***increase our profit per surgeon-hour?***" Exchanging $100 net per hour cosmetic services for $400+ net per hour classic ophthalmic care may be temporarily interesting if you're getting bored with geriatric ophthalmology, but it's a prescription for financial decline. In your own setting it may be better to beat a retreat today to the most profitable segments of eye care and leave behind a battle with dermatologists and boarded plastic surgeons that you can certainly wage, but are unlikely to win.

What other battles should you quit? Let's turn to low-profit and no-profit managed care contracts. These are signed innocently enough when you sense your clinic is not busy enough. (Have you ever noticed that contract signing time often coincides with those times of the year when practices are less busy?) After all, better to fill those empty appointment slots and enjoy a little marginal revenue, right? Wrong! Unless you're desperate for a near-term capital infusion, accepting ultra-low-fee and low-capitation contracts will only lull you into a sense of practice satiety, just like eating wood chips might give you a sense that you're well fed. Instead, such contracts devour the time needed to improve service quality and to plan and execute the marketing and outreach necessary to attract, over time, a higher-yielding patient base.

You should also retreat from the people who are wrong for your practice. Think to yourself: Do we have any lay staff or associate doctors who should be terminated today? If so, how long ago should they have left the practice? Why have we kept them so long? The same question set applies to your fellow practice partners. Should you keep up appearances—or worse yet, the heat of battle—or retreat from a partnership that isn't working? If you are an employee in an unwholesome setting, should you be quitting the battlefield your practice has become?

Continuing down the evacuation list, have you been putting off abandoning equipment that no longer works properly or should be replaced by a more profitable or clinically appropriate alternative? Are you maintaining unprofitable satellite offices—maybe branch offices that worked a decade ago when you were more energetic or worked for higher fees, but are now personally exhausting or uneconomic?

Should you retreat from surgical or clinical procedures that you personally do not do all that well or have not kept up with? Are there business procedures your staff now do more by rote, from outdated standing orders, than for any practice benefit? Are you still gathering financial or volume performance data that you're no longer using to make management decisions?

Ponder each of these questions, not in the abstract, but as they apply to your specific setting.

Are you doing things for yourselves within the practice, like payroll administration or office cleaning, that a vendor really could do better and cheaper? On the flip side, has your practice become laden with an overabundance of vendors who are performing functions better left to internal staff? Go through your general ledger, vendor by vendor, and give each one a score for necessity and another score for job performance and value.

Finally, and most broadly, is it time to drastically change your professional context? Is it time to be leaving the academic world for private practice, or vice versa? Is it time to stop your surgical career or leave medicine altogether?

• • •

Is it OK to quit? In some cases, no matter how foreign "giving up" is to the average eye surgeon, the answer is "absolutely." By confronting these difficult questions—and achieving a better life and practice with a little well-timed subtraction and backtracking—you'll be more inclined to win, like General Washington, over the long run.

Of Strategic Business Planning

Roald Amundsen, who was the first to lead a team to the South Pole, said, "Adventure is just bad planning." So, let's ask the question: Does your practice feel more like a wild adventure or more like a well-ordered expedition? How well do you plan?

About the same percentage of eye surgeons make long-term personal plans for their lives as make long-term plans for their practices, which is to say just above 0%.

Why is this? Why do surgeons not plan more? Why do most practices float aimlessly, goalless from year to year?

- Is it because you were on such a determinant, externally driven scholastic path for so many years that you were deconditioned from thinking about the future? (Because it was preordained for you.)
- Is it because the future of medical economics is a bit murky, so you figure, "What's the point in planning?"
- Or is it because the hyperdetailed, in-the-moment ophthalmic mind is unaccustomed to longer time frames? Perhaps your comfortable cycle time is the few minutes separating patient 1 from patient 2, not the few decades separating graduation day from your eventual retirement.

Whatever the reason, most ophthalmic ***practices*** and most ophthalmic ***lives*** suffer from planning insufficiency. And the two are connected.

• • •

What stimulates planning, anyway? Generally speaking, fear and greed.

Let's cover "fear" first. What induces fear? Change, or at least the prospect of change. The depth and tempo of business planning (and plan revision) is driven by how fast conditions are changing.

While most surgeons perceive that their practice environment is fragile and changing very fast, the business of medicine moves at a glacial pace compared to most industries. Medicare fee cuts, rising regulatory hurdles, and related practice bogeymen are benign compared to the pace of change in most business spheres.

Imagine being the CEO of Blackberry with a smartphone market share of 37% in the United States just 3 years ago, and getting your clock cleaned by Apple and Samsung, so that you now own less than a sliver of the market and are bleeding cash. That kind of abrupt displacement doesn't happen very often in ophthalmology. As a result, most ophthalmologists do not have much of a fear-based incentive to plan ahead.

And how about "greed" ... or more genteelly "ambition," as a driver for planning? Certainly, you are unlikely to become an eye surgeon unless you are academically ambitious. But unlike industrialists, who are commonly driven at the outset of their careers by a personal desire for great wealth, most ophthalmologists are not especially financially driven (although most eventually become very well off). And most surgeons live well below their means. They possess a kind of "needs insufficiency disorder," which can make it hard for administrators to light a business planning fire under them.

What else inhibits the process of planning? A distaste for confrontation. Ophthalmologists can be notoriously conflict adverse, which works against planning, at least in a group context, because planning obliges confrontation in the good and utilitarian sense of that word.

- Harry wants to grow the practice.
- Sue likes the practice just as it is.
- Mike is overwhelmed and would like to shrink back to the way things were.

These differences are important to work out, but eye surgeons are generally conflict-avoidant. So, sitting down around the table and coming up with a plan for the long-term future doesn't always come naturally.

• • •

All of this should not be taken as an excuse for not planning. Change ***is*** accelerating. There ***is*** more to rationally fear in the future environment. But, happily for the most ambitious surgeons reading this, there is also more opportunity than ever before to build a practice that is both clinically vanguard and commercially robust. There are more high-income eye surgeons today than at any time in the past.

Here are a few pearls to kick-start longer-term planning in your practice:

1. *All business strategic planning starts with personal planning.* I once had a confused client in his 50s, with a net worth vastly greater than his lifetime needs, and who no longer enjoyed medicine. He said he hired me for advice on how to ***build*** an even larger practice. This assignment quickly pivoted to helping this surgeon retire and divest his practice to a local colleague. As the saying goes, all business is personal. That goes double for eye care. Make sure that you are clear about your longer-term personal goals or your business planning will lead to creating an organization that is at odds with your life.
2. *Know the environment.* In most markets, your practice is no longer an island. What you will be able to build and add in the future (eg, satellites, specialty services, ancillary care) will depend on increasingly fragile access to patients. In the years ahead, some of you reading this will be locked out of access to new forms of managed care patient populations. Meet with every local hospital administrator and ask about the future of the local health care market.
3. *Be realistic about your skills.* Add complementary resources. You're probably a terrific surgeon. It is less likely that you are a great accountant, lawyer, or marketer. If your ambitions are high, draft proportionate resources.
4. *Perfect the core of the profession.* Your practice is not Ford Motor Company. As you walk from one exam room to the next you are personally creating and selling service-value units to one patient at a time. Five hundred great patient visits a month makes for a great practice. Do not try to expand until you can get the basics right.
5. *Strategic planning is a dynamic process.* The first draft of your plan is just a start. Your plan should be a live document, updated often.
6. *Answer eight simple questions about the years ahead:*
    - What is our natural service area?
    - What services will we add or subtract?
    - What's our positioning—what will we be known as? The discount practice? The most costly offering in our market? The managed care practice?
    - What will be our provider mix—what should be the ophthalmologist-to-optometrist ratio?
    - What will be our relationship to local institutions? Can we remain "Swiss," or must we link up with one health system or another?

- How fast will we aim to grow? Growing 4% to 5% per year will preserve our market share; growing faster will boost our market share, but can lead to operational hiccups.
- What ancillary services can we add to counter stagnant professional fees and rising operating costs?
- What will be my succession plan? How will I exit and recoup my investment?

• • •

The formal process of nominating a strategic plan for your practice will force you to see that practice and personal ambitions are entwined. The deliberate act of strategic planning, after years of random development, usually brings up insights beyond the question: Where am I taking my business? For thoughtful surgeons who are ready, the context broadens to: Where am I taking my life?

CHAPTER 4

Adaptability

There is no comparison between that which is lost by not succeeding and that which is lost by not trying.
—Sir Francis Bacon

Of Ophthalmology Then and Now

In just a single ophthalmic career span, 30 years or so, the American landscape has changed greatly—and eye care along with it. The current, logarithmic pace of change has been accelerated not just by the happy baseline of better technology and a more advanced civilization.

Whether you are personally at the front, back, or middle of your own career span, the change has been breathtaking. This is just a partial list of familiar things that have already slipped away or will in the coming years:

- Incandescent light bulbs
- Planned extracaps as the dominant surgical approach

Pinto JB. *Simple: The Inner Game of Ophthalmic Practice Success, Second Edition* (pp 43-63).

- VCR players
- $7-an-hour receptionists
- Printed phone books
- $5 to generate a prospective refractive surgery patient
- Film cameras (and nondigital angiography)
- Ophthalmologists denigrating optometrists, and vice versa
- Once-famous companies such as RCA, TWA, and Woolworth's
- Having to say, "What's better, one or 2?"
- Fifty-cent candy bars
- Ledger cards and Safeguard accounting systems
- $2 gasoline
- "Normal" 50% ophthalmic practice profit margins

For young doctors and managers who weren't around then, and for older ones who can't quite remember, here's an abstract of the 30-year before and after:

	Then...	...and Now
Capital outlays to reasonably equip a solo practice with contemporary equipment	Under $200,000	Over $500,000
First-year start-up costs for refractive surgery (eg, facilities, equipment, promotion)	About $150,000	About $1 million
Typical general ophthalmology practice profit margins (ie, percent of practice collections available for provider compensation)	40% to 50%	25% to 40%
Typical physician time spent on administration per week	About an hour	More than 5 hours
Goodwill value of a practice sold between doctors	About 50% of annual collections	50% or less of annual profits
Lay staffing costs as a percent of collections in a general ophthalmology practice	22% to 28%	28% to 33%
Core competencies for an effective practice manager	Billing skills and knowledge of basic clinical services	Robust financial, human resources, legal, regulatory, and marketing skills
Annual salary to employ a practice manager for a typical solo practice	$40,000	$70,000+
Computer system acquisition costs for a typical solo practice	Under $35,000	$50,000 to $150,000

As a result of these changes, the ophthalmology practice failure rate is rising. There is no national registry for ophthalmic bankruptcy, but my phone lines are a reasonable proxy. Thirty years ago, even 10 years ago, virtually all new client calls could be boiled down to: "We're doing great … can we do better?"

It's increasingly common to hear this instead from at least a third of my callers: "For the first time ever we're having a real challenge making payroll or meeting other practice expenses." Or in the apoplectic words of one delightfully crusty, senior ophthalmologist I know who practices with his young son, "My parking lot is empty! What the hell is going on?!?"

The short answer to the gentleman's question is the following:

- With 50% profit margins and limited competition a generation ago, ophthalmologists and their managers could almost run their businesses blindfolded.
- Until recently, you could make a lot of mistakes in a 35% margin and higher business and still do okay.
- Today, so-so managers and practice owners (even if they are great doctors), and those working in costly or overly competitive markets, are beginning to go under.
- Lower profit margins are unmasking errors in business judgment and gaps in operations that were previously occult. (As Warren Buffett said, "It's only when the tide goes out that you learn who's been swimming naked.") The most vulnerable 25% of ophthalmic practices in business today can be expected to either fail or be forced into the arms of a merger/acquisition partner in the years ahead.
- How well is your practice coping with these changes? How are ***you*** coping? Most of the problems ahead can be solved if you simply have access to enough patients; time to think; and enthusiastic, engaged providers and staff.

Here is a list of eight supplemental "survive and thrive" tactics:

1. *Continuous staff right-sizing and right-costing.* Support staff are the largest and most elastic cost element in your practice. If you have an up-and-down practice, you need to have up-and-down staffing levels. While you may think it is kindness to keep everyone at their promised 40 hours per week instead of floating staff to fewer hours in slow weeks, ask the staff you might have to terminate a few months from now because of your generosity. Be a leader. Protect the company. Hold the line.
2. *Abandon unprofitable enterprises.* If your low-volume LASIK practice, cosmetics services, or satellite office is breaking even or worse today, tomorrow will not be a better day in the current environment. Muster the discipline and the courage to discontinue unprofitable service lines and satellites. Redeploy your resources to more promising areas or trim them altogether.
3. *Provide ancillary services.* This includes employee providers, ASC facilities, and optical dispensing. If your surgeons are booked out several weeks and still providing lots of primary eye care, their time to serve secondary and tertiary patients should be expanded with optometric providers. If your state (like most) freely allows the development of private surgery centers, and you perform more than 50 major cases a month, then launch your own center. If you have a small optical that is run as a break-even patient convenience, turn it into a real business.

4. *Go where your services are needed.* If you still have a choice, steer clear of overly competitive markets. If you work in a community with fewer than 20,000 people per ophthalmologist, find outlying, underserved satellite opportunities to hedge against growing urban competition and provider contract shut-outs.
5. *Discipline with both business and personal expenses.* The most difficult client settings I consult in are those where cost structures—business, personal, or both—have been locked in without any advance "What if?" thinking. It's perfectly okay to splurge on great staff lunches or great vacations, which are nonrecurring costs you can pare instantly as needed. But it can paralyze you or your business to sign a 10-year lease for more space than you need or to buy a third vacation home on the strength of just one good year.
6. *Do more work.* Some ophthalmologists gasp at any more than 350 patient visits in a full month. Some surgeons I know lope along happily seeing that many patients in a long week. If your location or reputation has blessed you with an abundance of patients, harness this to stay several steps ahead of your less-fortunate colleagues. Also, reconsider your retirement timeline. Depending on how you have deployed your assets, you may need to push back your retirement date, your lifestyle in retirement, or both.
7. *Hire, train, and reward high-output staff.* Some techs can accurately work up a patient in 12 minutes. Some take 25 minutes, leave a wake of errors, and yet enjoy the same wages as the speedy worker. Identify and reward your most productive staff. Replace all of the rest. Train avidly, providing at least 1 hour of formal training for every 80-hour pay period.
8. *A survivalist's mindset.* When conditions change for the worse, some people are dispirited while others are energized. Try to be the second kind of person. If you were stranded in the wilderness, you would quickly go feral—learning to make fire, eat bugs, and sleep under the stars. Or you would die. We're happily nowhere near that point in eye care. But the foreseeable era is a time to abandon your assumptions about what you would or would not do to help your practice survive and thrive in the environment that lies ahead.

Of Sustainability

We're hearing a lot about sustainability—or rather ***un***sustainability—lately:

- Unsustainable ecology and climate
- Unsustainable energy resources
- Unsustainable housing bubbles
- Unsustainable federal deficits
- Unsustainable health care costs

Closer to home, at the level of managing your practice enterprise, we have an abundance of obviously unsustainable elements, and suspicions that more could be sneaking around the corner soon, such as:

- Unsustainable proliferation of new business, clinical, and surgical maneuvers to master each year
- Unsustainable rash of new regulations to follow
- Unsustainable time poverty for providers, whose work–life balance has evaporated
- Unsustainable economic pressures to be able to preserve high-quality care
- Unsustainable practice cost inflation
- Unsustainably small practices that will have to grow larger to survive

Most surgeons and their managers are tossed in a storm composed of this latter list of unsustainable practice elements, while a few are sailing along comfortably, confidently, and in control.

What's the key to this control and the peace of mind that comes with it? It is simple, really. You just need to apply the old familiar wisdom of changing the things you can, living with the things you can't, and knowing the difference between them. Here are some examples in the three critical domains of your practice: the macro/national environment, your practice's business environment, and in your personal financial circumstances. In each of these three areas you can have successively more personal control over sustainable outcomes.

Sustainable National Economics

This one is obviously the most unpleasant monster in the closet. Because of circumstances entirely out of your control (unless you are willing to emigrate) you happen to be a highly productive, law-abiding, tax-paying citizen of a country that is technically, if not practically—for the moment—bankrupt.

If you're like most intellectually honest eye surgeons, you're probably of dual minds about this. Half of your brain wants the federal government to get its act together, live within its means, and especially trim entitlement spending, which is the most unsustainable rump of our federal deficit spending problem. And half of your brain is scared that Washington might actually do all of this and more—perhaps devastatingly clipping your financial wings for life.

The average ophthalmologist depends on the sustainability and predictability of federal and state entitlement spending for more than 60% of practice cash flow. Even the ultimately benign, serially withdrawn threats of fee cuts over the past several years are enough to induce profound provider anxiety and put a crimp on business planning, practice succession transactions, and hiring.

The only sound mitigation advice here, since you have almost no practical personal influence over what happens in the nation's capital, is the following:

- Stay as informed as you can. Reading widely will help you peer around corners and better make (or forego) investments in your business.
- Write a "20+% Disaster Plan." Right now, you probably have a sense of generalized anxiety about how you would respond to a deep cut in fees. Combat these feelings with a spreadsheet. What costs would you curtail? Would you be able to increase appointment slots and find patients to fill them? Could you take in a compatible local colleague and share costs and cross-referrals? What would you have left to live on? Could you do it?

- Stay involved through your professional societies with lobbying and advocacy fundraising efforts. Just as your sole individual vote has no material influence on who wins your local mayoral race, your efforts federally are an even more diluted drop in the ocean. But acting collectively is your duty as a national and ophthalmologic citizen, and will afford you some finite sense of involvement. At the very least, you'll have a right to complain about what happens next.

Sustainable Practice Economics

Now we are entering a domain where you have a little more control—but only within limits. You might be thinking, "Well, I'm not worried. If they cut my fees, I'll just cut salaries across the board and tell my landlord they have to take a hit with me." That may work in a few markets. But for the rest of the country, you're going to be competing with other, nonmedical employers for staff and nonmedical tenants for office space. Like as not, you'll have to pay market rates for both.

Sustainability at a practice level is not so much about cutting this or that ***cost,*** but having a global awareness of about 50 or so key business "dashboard" items, so you'll always know when you're safe and when a crash is imminent. These benchmarks have been widely published (many of my books have them), and there's no longer any excuse to be in the dark about practice performance.

Still, it is shocking to see how many practices are still driving blind.

I know the administrator of a $2 million practice who only generates a financial statement quarterly and couldn't quote the profit margin of her practice. Her doctors know even less about the business. That's the kind of practice that keeps consultants awake at night.

Sustainable Personal Economics

This is where you have the most control and the greatest ability to create a sustainable environment. The most fortunate eye surgeons—and happily still the majority—live on a lot less than they earn. It is hard to spend money when you work 60 hours a week, which leads to ample savings and a secure retirement. However, a slowly growing minority of surgeons are reporting to me that they are living on 100% or more of their earnings.

This is a problem whether you earn $100,000 and spend $101,000, or make a million and spend a million and one dollars. It's all the same kind of misery. In a study a colleague and I conducted of surgeon happiness and satisfaction, the happiest surgeons live on the lowest percentages of their income.

If you're veering toward a personal budgetary crisis, it's more important than ever before that you take brisk, assertive steps to change direction. There are at least two reasons for this. First, because ophthalmic incomes are likely to continue to soften, you want to get out ahead of any gaps between income and outgo. And second, because the accumulation of retirement savings is expected to be tougher for the next generation or longer, with lower rates of capital appreciation, higher inflation, and higher tax rates.

These assertive steps should include the following:

- Engage your accountant or hire a fee-only personal financial planner to help you plan for the future (and if you like to manage your own financial affairs, at the very least get a periodic second opinion from a professional).
- Review your trajectory to retirement. Numerous quick-and-dirty programs are available online, but that's just a crude starting point for a more thoroughgoing review and plan.
- Live on 80% or less of your income—if you want to preserve your current lifestyle in retirement and are saving less than 20% of your total earnings, it is unlikely you are putting funds away at a fast-enough pace.
- It may be necessary to cut lifestyle costs. Benchmark personal expenditures in every category for the last year (ie, like a profit and loss statement for your practice) and hold a family meeting to agree on new expenditure targets. If necessary, use external sources of discipline, such as your planner or accountant, to keep you from straying from the plan.

• • •

Just as in surgery, a successful life is all about planning and control. Gone are the luxuriant days when so much revenue sloshed around in eye care—a time when there was always enough money to buy your way out of trouble or start over again. Adopt a philosophy of sustainability in every area under your control—and back that philosophy up with ***action.***

Of Disaster Planning

For all of the country's preoccupation with "homeland security," precious little attention is paid by ophthalmic practice owners to the far greater odds of a personal, professional, or natural disaster striking your business. It's not very likely that terrorists are going to knock you out of business. But a majority of surgeons will experience at least one of the common knockout punches thrown by fate. With a little advance contingency planning, you can duck or block the worst of these.

Let's examine the most common disasters and what you can do to blunt their impact on your practice, your earnings, and, perhaps most importantly, your peace of mind.

• • •

Personal health problems clearly top the calamity list. It's hard to get through 30+ years of an ophthalmic career without at least one or two health-related work interruptions—either to yourself personally, a member of your family, or a key member of your staff. A skiing accident may knock out production for just a few predictable weeks. Bigger health problems may leave you permanently disabled. If your practice and family are depending on you, you need to prepare for the worst.

To the extent you can control your medical destiny through good habits, stay healthy. Most eye surgeons are fairly fit, given the aerobics of walking from room to room throughout the day. A little extra exercise, along with dietary wisdom and stress relief, will forestall most health-related workplace disruptions and pay dividends in greater energy every day. Middle-aged clients commonly report that a modest exercise program will reset their biological clock back a decade, increase output, and reduce the stress of modern practice.

Make sure you are adequately insured, not only for the treatment of an acute medical crisis but for a chronic partial or full disability. These policies are increasingly costly and constrictive, as insurers have learned that doctors are particularly clever at feigning a disability. Therefore, at some point a degree of self-insurance is obliged, especially to cover the early months of a disability. Set funds aside—personally or corporately—to bridge the typical delay until disability or business interruption insurance kicks in.

Money is the universal solvent for most practice flutters. It can't bring a permanently disabled partner back to work, or immediately restore a flooded building, but money buys time to wait the problem out or start all over again.

Every practice should have an open line of credit equal to at least 3 months of core expenses. If it costs $150,000 per month for the largely fixed staff, facility, equipment lease, and similar costs in your practice, you should have $450,000 or more at the ready. This can be a combination of personal savings, a line of credit, receivables, and working bank accounts.

One of the toughest decisions faced by doctors in disasters is whether to stick it out and rebuild or move on. I had clients in both categories after Hurricane Katrina, and I've also been involved in tough judgment calls related to medical emergencies.

I recall one of these on the Eastern seaboard. An intense, successful solo surgeon in his forties suffered a stroke. In the initial weeks, he, his physicians, and his family believed he would be able to return to work—at least in some capacity—within a matter of months. The months dragged on. And on. Rather than selling the practice briskly, the family hired a locum physician to try to keep the practice going.

In the end, this unfortunate surgeon was obliged to retire. And his practice? Other surgeons in the region picked off enough of it that within a year there was nothing left to sell but the tangibles, which went for salvage value. In hindsight, it would have been wiser to engage a local, competing doctor as the putative buyer at the outset of the stroke and execute a purchase option agreement in case the disabled surgeon was unable to return to work.

Here are a few additional common disasters, large and small, and steps you can take to blunt them.

Loss of Key Personnel

Smaller practices are amazingly susceptible to the loss of key staff members. In the typical solo practice, just one person knows the computer system and billing protocols. The surgeon-owners in such settings are obliged to become co-key operators of their information systems and to also be fluent in patient accounts management. With rare exceptions, soloists ***must*** know how to post a charge, submit claims, and run routine system reports—or be held hostage by a key employee. Beyond this, in all settings large and small, redundancy is key. It's wonderful to have a superstar administrator, but make sure that your practice's mid-level management team is sufficiently cross-trained to be able to cover the majority of your administrator's duties if disaster strikes.

Embezzlement

Although awareness and monitoring have increased in the past generation, embezzlement is still a common occurrence. Your accounting firm should have a regular (and highly visible) spot audit protocol in place, partly to detect any diversion, but mostly to reduce staff temptations. Bonding can add to your peace of mind, as can criminal background checks of all new hires. Deep reference checks should be obliged for all key hires.

A "Mono-Culture" Practice

Wise farmers grow a lot of different crops—if plant disease or adverse weather conditions arise, they can still survive. In the same way, wise eye surgeons avoid an overdependence on any single procedure, especially volatile procedures such as LASIK or elective plastics. If you are unable or unwilling to diversify, then at least sequester the funds needed to weather any anticipated reversals. In LASIK, it is common for national recessions or adverse local economic news to kill practice profits ... and this can continue for several quarters. Dedicated refractive surgeons should develop capital and treasury policies, giving them access to a year or more of core practice costs and personal living expenses.

Lack of Facility Redundancy

Severe weather-related disasters in recent years have shown a number of eye surgeons the wisdom of maintaining multiple offices, as well as second homes. In one client's case, three out of four office buildings were destroyed in New Orleans, but a fourth office survived, providing a kind of practice "life raft." In other cases, surgeons were able to easily retreat from a shattered New Orleans to their second homes out of state. (Here's the excuse you've been looking for to buy that ski condo or New York apartment you've always wanted!)

Divorce

Some disasters transcend anything that Mother Nature can throw your way. For ophthalmologists who divorce, a number of underlying business challenges go beyond the obvious personal difficulties. If the dissolution goes poorly, dispirited eye surgeons will typically enter a period of 1 year or longer of reduced productivity due to legal distractions and financial resentments. Prevention is vastly preferable to curing marital strife, of course. But, it's difficult to choose a partner during your training years (as typically happens) and then sustain this relationship in the wake of profoundly changing financial, professional, and family circumstances. This can be compounded in increasingly common doctor–doctor marriages. Resort to professional counseling at the first sign of discord. The best defensive, if unromantic, solution is a prenuptial agreement spelling out augmented financial and other practice rights in the event of divorce.

Malpractice Suits

Welcome to America. Beyond extreme caution, defensive medicine, and kindness, your only resort in the face of legal challenges is to choose to practice in favorable states and insure to the hilt. But you do have a measure of control. With rare exceptions, patients sue more often due to bad relationships than bad outcomes. You must either be a perfect practitioner, learn how to delight patients, or steer clear of those elective procedures that are most often prosecuted. Follow your instincts (and the instincts of staff) and refer unreasonable patients out of your practice.

Unwise Actions by Fellow Doctors

Not only do you have to mind your own behavior … you have to worry about the actions of your colleagues. Experience shows that a majority of group practices will be damaged sooner or later by the adverse behaviors of one or more partners or associates. These behaviors include substance abuse, sexual harassment, reckless medical care, and billing fraud. There are five essential safeguards for organizations and their leaders:

1. *Select doctors carefully.* It is very difficult to effectively screen for untoward behaviors and frank antisocial tendencies. MMPI and similar psychological testing instruments are favored in some settings—but trust your instincts above all else.
2. *Write employment contracts that place the consequences squarely on the offending doctor.* It is common for practices to outlay initial funds to defend harassment, fraud, and similar suits. Subject to the input of your attorney, doctor employment contracts should specify that the culpable doctors are responsible for reimbursing these costs and holding their fellow providers harmless.
3. *Establish and follow firm policies.* Turn to your attorney for assistance; this is now largely boilerplate. Realize that your general business attorney may not have the necessary experience to deal with Medicare fraud or sexual harassment issues—retain subspecialty counsel where indicated.
4. *Monitor behaviors.* Training and consciousness raising is not enough; I have been in practices where the doctors are obliged to sign off after every yearly refresher training, but that still have trouble with rampant harassment.
5. *Pounce vigorously on offenses.* Foster a consequential environment—the practice's MP is unfortunately cast in the role of cop to intervene with offending colleagues. When they are the offender, the board has to step in, of course.

Adverse Payer Audits

We can expect deeper levels of provider scrutiny in the years ahead, particularly if electronic medical records and pay-for-performance systems create more seamless and automatic oversight by payers. Retain the services of a charting, billing, and coding consultant and develop a compliance plan. In the end, knowing precisely where the line is drawn can help you optimize reimbursement. Brace yourself for the day when highly specific care pathways are not just "preferred" but obliged.

Computer Woes

Back in the quaint, old days of individual patient ledger cards and paper claims, the only system "crash" you needed to hedge against was running out of ink in your pen. Today, your practice's cash flow hangs by a thin silicon thread. Thankfully, today's systems are so reliable that we tend to overlook this vulnerability. But, even if your practice's computer system is flawless (and none are), you are still susceptible to payer system flaws. Doctors have experienced months-long interruptions in cash flow from Medicare associated with carrier computer conversions gone awry. This is one more reason to have a credit line in place before you need it.

A Lack of Connections

In my experience, most eye surgeons are fiercely independent souls, not given to developing wide networks of friends who can rally to their assistance. But this isn't always the case. I remember a well-loved eye doctor in North Carolina who was in a terrible auto accident. Although he didn't have any kind of formal agreement with his local competitors, they took turns covering his solo practice for several months, turning over 100% of the billings, until he could return to work 6 months later. Larger group practices can and commonly do internally self-insure in this fashion. Looking beyond your own town, keep up contacts in the national community—you may need to call them for a job one day when the next 9/11 or Katrina hits.

• • •

To sum it up, assume the best but prepare for the worst. Have a written disaster plan. Let your key staff, partners, and family know what you would like done in the event of your incapacitation. Which advisors should be contacted to give staff and family advice about sustaining, winding down, or selling the practice? If you can no longer practice, who in the community would you like to take over your patient base?

Of Entrepreneurism

Entrepreneurism is the positive counterpart of mere business survival. Entrepreneurs most often arise in the presence of adversity. They see opportunity where others see doom.

Lots of people are called "entrepreneurs," from the kid at the end of your street selling lemonade to Jeff Bezos. And if you're an ophthalmologist running your own practice, you probably think you qualify as an entrepreneur. But are you really?

What defines a doctor-entrepreneur? Is it starting a solo practice on your own? Taking over a small practice and making it larger? Adding a new elective procedure and handling all the details from service development to promotion and pricing? These are all vanguard activities that would make you stand out from the crowd of eye surgeons who take a safer path. And these are certainly examples of "little-e" entrepreneurism.

But to my way of thinking, to be a "BIG-E" Entrepreneur, you need to take your business enterprise to the next step: from a business that lives and dies based on your personal, daily inputs—to an enterprise that no longer needs your daily production or presence.

Here's a simple self-exam to determine if you're a "BIG-E" or "little-e" entrepreneur, or if you might be better suited to join an existing enterprise rather than struggling to build one of your own. There is no value judgment in this exam; it's equally honorable to score high or low.

Vision and Opportunism

Doctors at every place in the entrepreneurial spectrum can creatively take in the facts and data of their business environment, dream about the future, and invent in great detail the endpoint they then aim for. Which of these three attributes best fits you?

____ 1. People who know me well often kid me about how I have my head in the clouds. I really enjoy imaging my practice in the distant future and am very comfortable thinking in terms of a 5-, 10-, even 20-year plan. I really do not mind if it turns out that my long-term vision was incorrect—I just really need a big goal to strive for. When I see a clinical or business trend, I'm often among the first to jump on it. ***(5 points)***

____ 2. I can readily think of my practice in terms of 3 to 5 years out, but beyond that the picture gets fuzzy. I do not think we can reliably predict the environment any farther ahead than that, and I'd rather not get my hopes up for nothing. I'm neither the first nor the last person to adopt new ideas and trends. ***(3 points)***

____ 3. I prefer to wake up and simply take each day as it comes. I've never really been one to plan my life or career out more than the next year. When I see a new trend, I like to wait to see how it pans out, and not be the first one to jump in ... it might just be a fad. ***(1 point)***

Positive Versus Negative Orientation

Super-entrepreneurs tend to be extremely positive people. They see the glass as half full and believe that even the most difficult circumstances will somehow lead to an otherwise undiscovered opportunity.

____ 1. I have found that life pretty much gives you what you can handle and overcome—even the toughest breaks. I may get down from time to time when disappointments arise, but this feeling is fleeting, and I bounce back stronger than ever. I mostly wear a smile, even at times when most people would be down. My staff are attracted to my positive outlook on life, and I really enjoy getting folks to see the bright side whenever problems come up. ***(5 points)***

_____ 2. I am a realist. So, when problems come up in the practice, I groan like the next person. However, for the sake of the team, I put on a smile when I must, even if down deep I'm really worried and pessimistic. I do appreciate being around "up" people who can keep me from thinking the cup is half empty. ***(3 points)***

_____ 3. I believe that life is basically difficult and unfair, unless you happen to be one of the few people who get lucky. It really bugs me to be around highly optimistic, positive people—I mean, who's kidding whom? Life's tough. Keep a low profile, be careful, and you won't get hurt. ***(1 point)***

Ability to Drive to the Finish

All the business brilliance in the world has to be combined with years and years of hard work to see your plans come to life. Each of these years contains an opportunity to throw your hands up and quit pressing so hard. Giving up prematurely on a satellite, an associate doctor, or a marketing plan is a lot easier than gutting it out and making things work. Strong entrepreneurs keep marching forward when others would quit. Which of these following three options best describes you?

_____ 1. When a project is looking dim, that's when I really shine. I just can't bear the thought of quitting something our practice has made a commitment to accomplish. My clinical and business career is full of examples where pushing just a little harder and longer, no matter the cost, gets the job done. ***(5 points)***

_____ 2. When I'm faced with adversity I'll push for a while, but not like some people I know. I'm all for giving projects our best shot, but when it seems we might be going in the wrong direction, I change course pretty quickly. ***(3 points)***

_____ 3. When projects get tough, that's a clear signal to me that it's time to quit. There's only so much we can do, and if we take on too much, we're going to fail. It doesn't take much for me to say, "Let's try something else, this isn't working." ***(1 point)***

Risk Taking

Some of us love risk, others are risk-adverse. Most are between these two extremes. The classic entrepreneur will mortgage their home to start a long-shot business. Risk must obviously be weighed by an intelligent judgment of the odds involved, the consequences of failure, and the scale of offsetting benefits.

_____ 1. I *love* taking calculated risks. So long as the odds are even remotely in our favor, and the potential payoff is big, I'll roll the dice and go for it. If it's legal and ethical, and the potential payoff is large, I'd risk almost anything if it could help us accomplish my long-term dreams. ***(5 points)***

_____ 2. I do not feel comfortable putting it all on the line, but I'm OK proceeding with policies and projects for the practice that we can reasonably survive in the event of failure. ***(3 points)***

_____ 3. I break out in a cold sweat and my heart races just *thinking* about taking a business or clinical risk. ***(1 point)***

Delegation

This is one of the most important attributes of any entrepreneur, but especially in medicine, where it's common to say, "It's faster to do this myself." Unlike a car wash or furniture store, it's much harder to build an ophthalmology practice and turn it over to non-owner employees to run for you and generate a passive profit. But that's exactly what the entrepreneurial doctors of the future will be doing.

_____ 1. Anything that others can do for me, I delegate avidly. That goes for clinical, surgical, and business chores. I know that if I would simply stop and take 30 minutes to teach someone a task, I can potentially save myself hundreds of hours over the course of the next few years. ***(5 points)***

_____ 2. I am pretty good at delegation, but still find myself from time to time doing routine, mundane tasks that others in the practice could be handling for me. ***(3 points)***

_____ 3. Nobody can do things as well as I can, so I rarely delegate. ***(1 point)***

Business Versus Practice Orientation

Some practices run their operations like a 1970s nonprofit foundation, with little regard for the bottom line and every decision based solely on the quality of care. Other (thankfully few) practices are on the opposite side of the spectrum, ignoring quality in the interest of profits. Over the last 2 decades, it has been increasingly necessary to shift somewhat from a "foundational" model to a "bottom line" model. Just where you place yourself on this continuum is obviously a sensitive and difficult decision for every eye surgeon today.

_____ 1. I absolutely respect and honor my role as a clinician, providing the very best care I can to my patients. But having said that, I know in today's world you have to run an ophthalmology practice like a business, and that's exactly what we do. ***(5 points)***

_____ 2. I would say that an increasing number of our decisions are driven by the bottom line, but that still leaves us running things kind of casually around here. ***(3 points)***

_____ 3. Even at the risk of business failure, I run my practice the old-fashioned way, and I'm not about to change. ***(1 point)***

Reproducible "Systems" Thinking

Medicine is both an art and a science, and a great deal of spirited discussion is now playing out about what the balance should be between the two of these. Scaling up, training extenders, and delegating requires that entrepreneurs take a systematic approach to care ... doing things the same, predictable way each time to the extent possible.

____ 1. I think of our practice as a finely tuned assembly line, in the good sense of that concept. We try to break down every step of the patient visit, and have it go as predictably, smoothly, briskly, and pleasantly for the patient as we can. Everyone here knows our practice's agreed "best way" to do just about everything. ***(5 points)***

____ 2. I have made this practice a little more systematic and organized than most, but I allow our doctors and staff a wide degree of latitude in how they care for patients. ***(3 points)***

____ 3. We are clinical artists. I treat each patient encounter as a highly customized event, based on the patient's personality and their unique needs. We really do not think in terms of "care pathways," "branching logic trees," or "algorithms"—we just take care of every patient based on what seems to be right for them at the time. ***(1 point)***

Process Documentation and Control

Let's compare professional surgeons to professional airline pilots. Somewhere long ago you read a cataract textbook or two enumerating the step-by-step process of safe and effective surgery. But the odds are very small, after of thousands of cases, that you have anything like a how-to checklist for surgery today, because it's all become a rote routine for you. And the pilot? There are manuals and checklists galore, even after thousands of hours logged in the air. Medicare, at least for now, is a lot looser than the FAA, obviously. And this same laxity resonates to your practice's business operations, unless—as an entrepreneur—you've recognized the value of process documentation and controls. Which of these following three options best describes you?

____ 1. I have insisted that we prepare and regularly update an operations manual for the practice. This is used for training, procedure auditing, and regular staff recredentialing. ***(5 points)***

____ 2. Many of our important procedures are written down, but at least half of what staff members do is in their heads and passed on verbally to new staff members. ***(3 points)***

____ 3. We only have a few handwritten crib notes, the rest of what we do is not documented in any way. ***(1 point)***

Staff Selection, Training, and Development

Being entrepreneurial and growing at faster rates requires that you replicate your ace technician's or billing clerk's skills down among the rest of the staff ranks, and that you do this efficiently and consistently—so that everyone is taking pressure checks and posting charges in the same, optimal way. To do otherwise results in error, frustration, and costly rework.

_____ 1. We put lots of time and care into perfecting systems here, so we only hire those workers who have a willingness and ability to learn our way of doing things. We quickly weed out new staff who can't step up to our pace, fit into our team mode, or who insist on importing the bad habits they learned at their last job. In fact, we're so good at spotting raw talent and "trainability," that we no longer rely on finding experienced staff—we grow our own experts, which saves us a lot in labor costs. ***(5 points)***

_____ 2. Of course, we think that staff selection and training are important, but frankly we're so overwhelmed with day-to-day patient care that we do not put much time into the hiring or training process. We follow our instincts, hire the best people we can find at the time, give them a week to settle in, then it's sink or swim. Lots of our new staff drown and leave well before their probation period is over. ***(3 points)***

_____ 3. We almost always hire staff who have experience from somewhere else and let them run with the way they've done things in their last job. It means we have to pay top dollar, and there's not that much consistency, but it makes life easier for our managers to not have to waste their time training workers from scratch. ***(1 point)***

Process Improvement

Even in the most successful, mature companies, constant and ongoing improvement is essential for continued prosperity. Every owner and manager—ideally every single member of the team—should be questioning every process and subroutine for opportunities to reduce costs or improve quality.

_____ 1. In our practice, there are no sacred cows and everything we do is subject to scrutiny. We not only do this formally by ourselves, but we invite patients, payers, visiting doctors and managers from other practices, consultants, and regulatory officials to tell us how to do a better job. We are not defensive when hearing criticism. And we do not just listen, we rapidly implement every reasonable suggestion. We see the job of "improving" like housework—something that is never finished. ***(5 points)***

_____ 2. From time to time we ask ourselves, "Could we do this or that better?" We read articles and go to national meetings, and frequently we'll find a pearl here or there. But you know, there's probably not that much more we could do to improve without driving everyone crazy. ***(3 points)***

____ 3. I guess we're pretty complacent around here. It takes a major clinical blunder or patient complaint for us to stand back as a team and reinvent the way we do things. We certainly do not go out of our way looking for outside advice. And even when we improve something, things often shift back to the way they were. Old habits are hard to break. ***(1 point)***

Fiscal Management and Resource Apportionment

In bygone days of 50+% profit margins, financial planning and cash flow management was relatively easy. There were plenty of reserves to fund any reasonable practice initiative. Today, ophthalmology is typically a ± 35% profit margin business. And we are on an all-but-inevitable glide path to the lower percentile levels seen in "normal" businesses. Business growth takes time, expertise, and capital. Lots and lots of capital.

____ 1. The doctors here realize that to grow we must invest profits back in the practice. To accomplish this, we have a lot of personal discipline. We have each learned how to sacrifice and live on a lot less than we make. We know that if we invest wisely, the practice will thrive. We may take a personal pay cut this month, and even this year, but we're confident that over the next 10 years, we'll be dollars ahead, provide better care, and be more secure in our market. ***(5 points)***

____ 2. Doctors in our practice take a middle path. We are certainly willing to fund obvious money-making opportunities, but the payback period had better be within the next year or we would just as soon take the money home personally. ***(3 points)***

____ 3. The doctors take every available penny out of the practice. Even though we've been in business for years and years, we're still caught short during lean months and have a hard time making payroll. Our facility is getting a little shabby. We're short of some equipment. It feels like we're starving the golden goose. ***(1 point)***

Succession Modeling, Planning, and Execution

Every individual ophthalmic ***career*** has a beginning, a middle, and a finite end. Not so ***practices,*** which with planning can live on, constantly improving and growing, for many generations. Some eye surgeons see their practices as a personal ATM machine, something they would just as soon discard at the end of their career rather than taking on the hassle and uncertainties of bringing in one or more successors. Other ophthalmologists think in bigger terms. They see their practices as institutions that should outlive them, serving future doctors, staff, and patients. Like proud and responsible parents, such doctors are more than willing to make personal sacrifices to see that their practices live on and succeed.

_____ 1. It would be a very great disappointment to me to not have my practice thrive and grow after I'm retired. To this end, I've already worked out a timeline for phasing in the next doctors. My plan even includes a way for me to earn a little passive income during the last years of my practice, and to have a private office to come to and work on my novel after I've retired from medicine. ***(5 points)***

_____ 2. It would be nice to see some young doctors carry on with my practice after I'm out of the picture, but if that comes at the cost and risk of taking on young associates who are a pain and might not work out, forget it. Maybe in the last 3 years of active practice I'll try to find a successor, but not at the cost of topping up my retirement savings. If it doesn't work out the first time, or maybe the second, I'll just work until I'm ready to walk away and hand the keys over to one of my local colleagues. ***(3 points)***

_____ 3. I see the business nuts and bolts of my practice as a personal tool to use so long as I'm professionally active, and then discard. I worked hard to build this practice with little help from anyone else. Let the next person figure it out for themselves. ***(1 point)***

• • •

Now add up your total score, and see where you seem to fit in the ranges below. The maximum score is 60, the minimum is 12.

50 to 60 points: Consider yourself a "BIG-E" Entrepreneur. You may have the drive, perspectives, and attitudes necessary to build a larger, multigenerational, multilocation, multisubspecialty practice that at some point in the future no longer needs your personal input. Such a business could provide you with a passive source of income or allow your personal take home pay to rise, even as fees and profit margins fall, by hiring employee providers to increase your practice's total output well beyond your individual capacity.

25 to 49 points: Perhaps you're a "little-e" entrepreneur, which is the vast majority of eye surgeons. You still want to build a great business, deliver outstanding care, and may even be successful in passing it on to successors who pay you a small buyout for what you have created. But nearly all of your income from the practice will be active—generated by your own personal efforts—not passive. As fees fall along with typical profit margins, and you reach the limits of your personal time and output, your income will inevitably fall.

Under 25 points: You may be more comfortable, happy, and successful in a modest practice, operating at relative stasis, where there is a lot of room for customization and complexities can be kept under your personal control. Alternately, as medical economics change and put a premium on efficiency and scale, it may be appropriate for you to consider joining a more entrepreneurial practice, rather than building a larger company on your own.

Please keep in mind that wherever you score on this informal self-evaluation is perfectly OK so long as you're true to your personality, your aspirations, and the practical realities of your local marketplace. And please realize that there's an important age-related factor in all of this. It's not at all unusual for doctors younger than 40 and older than 55 to be quite averse to being entrepreneurial, and doctors 40 to 55 to be more risk taking and progressive. It may be interesting for you to bring this evaluation tool out every few years to see how your perspectives change over time.

Of Adaptability

Sir William Osler, one of the great teachers of premodern medicine, said in an 1897 address to the New York Academy of Medicine, "When schemes are laid in advance, it is surprising how often the circumstances fit in with them." In other words, for success, plan your work—and then work your plan. It sounds like Osler was time-traveling to the present era.

Osler is better known for his famous quote: "Availability, affability, and ability are what young doctors need to build a practice. And, in that order of importance." Had he worked in today's fast-changing environment, he probably would have added a fourth "A" to the familiar medical student's 3-A axiom. He would have added "adaptability" and put it at the front of the list.

You should, too, in this weird, breath-holding era.

This moment in medical economics should be stimulating your instincts to loosen up and become more adaptable. Here are some practical things to keep you and your practice light on its feet and nimbly adapting to the world ahead for all of us.

• • •

First things first. The largest operating expense in every practice is lay staffing, so that's the first place to be braced and ready to take action. If, against all predictions, steep fee cuts do occur in the next few years—or indeed, if fees do not rise but inflation does—you may have no option but to trim staffing costs. Such cost-cutting can snip in numerous variations, large and small:

- Cutting the number of staff to transit a given volume of patients
- Cutting staff hours across the board to accomplish the same economic result
- Freezing or reducing wages—this could include eliminating annual cost-of-living allowances (replacing them with spot bonuses) or selective pay cuts
- Labor substitution—this can take many forms: replacing full-time staff with part-time to save benefits costs, replacing low-level adult clerks with casual labor from the local high school, eliminating tech positions and performing some of your own work-ups, and terminating underperforming associate providers (putting their patients on your own schedule)
- Outsourcing back-office business functions, such as billing, payroll, or human resources, which may be more costly for you to manage than send to an outside specialist

Most of these changes are painful to one degree or another, which gets to the heart of being "adaptable." You have to be able personally to accommodate to this kind of discomfort and be willing to confront tough decisions *with the interests of the practice placed ahead of any one individual, including yourself as a leader.* Not to press the survivor analogy too far, this is no different than a lost hiker adapting to their new situation by fighting back fear, drinking brackish water, and pushing their body to the edge of endurance.

Such unpleasant, even painful changes must of course be in line with the rest of your behavior as an owner. If the day arrives when you have to prescribe bitter medicine for the staff, you can't turn around and order a new luxury car, buy a nonessential clinical tool, or book an island cruise.

The second largest outlay—and a target for adaptation efforts—is for office facilities. There are several ways to increase adaptability in this area:

- Commit to shorter lease periods, and more liberal escape clauses, even if it might cost a bit more. This is especially the case for any facilities beyond your core location.
- Unless growth is highly ensured, err on the low side of how much space you will need.
- When opening up in a new area, lease office space until success in your own building is more ensured (of course, the catch-22 with this more cautious strategy is that by that time, land and building prices may have gone up).
- Rather than owning or leasing your own dedicated office, rent space (and staff) by the hour, day, or month from compatible colleagues who may also be in a position to refer patients to you.
- Be more circumspect in examining satellite office opportunities. Having two offices can be four times more complex than a single location and lead to operational mix-ups and lower profits in the original office.

Of course, enhancing bottom-line performance is more a matter of boosting revenue than containing costs. Remember that adding just ***one*** patient per clinic day can generate enough incremental revenue in a year to cover one staff member's salary and benefits—***2*** new patients per day and you come out ahead.

We are entering an era when the demand for services is rising, while fees are stagnant (and falling in real, inflation-adjusted terms). Now is the time to discover a few new personal "gears." If you have been operating two cases an hour, call the team together and shoot for 3. If you have a weeks-long backlog of patients and are topping out at 45 visits per day, take a field trip to a 60-patient-per-day colleague to see how it can be done.

Are you ready for what lies ahead? Here's a quiz that will test your own adaptability to the environment we may well be facing. If you can answer "Yes" to a majority of these five questions, you may already be sufficiently armored for the future:

1. Imagine that double-digit fee cuts are a reality. Your personal income will soon also drop by double digits. Are you the kind of person who could probably learn to live with this new reality and shift your source of satisfaction to other spheres?
2. Adapting means changing, and all change (even the good kind) is stressful. Would others say about you that you typically adapt well to stress and change?

3. Do you have a clever, inventive nature that makes you confident about operating an eye clinic in tougher circumstances? (A hint: If you have ever been on an overseas mission, that was a perfect test for this kind of ingenuity and ability to do more with less.)
4. You can't control the trajectory of fee reform, but you ***can*** control your ability to mitigate softer fees with harder work and seeing more patients every day. Do you possess the health and energy reserves that would allow you to ramp up your output?
5. If you work with partners, are your relationships with each other strong enough to endure any financial or other resource challenge anticipated in the years ahead?

CHAPTER 5

Metrics

If money be not thy servant, it will be thy master.
—Sir Francis Bacon

OF NUMERACY ... MASTERING MATH AS A SECOND LANGUAGE

Psychologist Sian Beilock at the University of Chicago explained to NBCNews.com why math is so uncomfortable for some people. Apparently, the mental anguish that math-adverse people feel is sourced to the same ancient, evolutionarily primitive area of our brains—the dorso-posterior insula—which is activated when we experience bodily, physical pain.

In math phobes, just the mere ***thought*** of having to do math is enough to light up this region of the brain. Of course, this research has important consequences in

Pinto JB. *Simple: The Inner Game of Ophthalmic Practice Success, Second Edition* (pp 65-99).

the sphere of practice administration, because the clearest dividing line between good and great administrators is their comfort with math.

I know scores of otherwise very bright OMs who have been stuck for years at a level barely above the level of clerk because of weak math skills. For them, math is a kind of impenetrable second language that they can't seem to learn. Just the act of trying to puzzle out a business-made problem hurts.

If you want to be a great ophthalmic business leader—and make the leap from "clerk" or "manager" to "administrator," it is essential that you learn to think like a doctor, which is to bravely engage with the world of objective facts and data.

Medicine, after all—particularly the ophthalmic kind—is largely about numbers.

- A refraction generates a numeric prescription.
- An intraocular pressure check yields two numbers.
- Even cataracts are graded on a numeric scale.

We are no longer in an environment like we had when I started consulting in ophthalmology more than 30 years ago. Back then, "Patient doing fine" was a perfectly acceptable and complete chart note. Back then, an equally subjective business performance report was also acceptable: "Billing is all caught up."

Everyone is at least a little bit anxious about math, just like we are all a little bit anxious about flying or public speaking, no matter how much of it we do. That is normal. But practice administrators who are truly math phobic are as held back in their careers as are administrators who can't stand up in front of the staff to give a training session or fly to a national symposium.

Experts say that severe phobia is a learned anxiety. No one is born afraid of flying or speaking or doing math. Your dislike for math is probably rooted in a belittling teacher or parent. Nearly all of us over a certain age have had the experience of being called up to the blackboard to solve a math problem with our classmates looking on. (For some of you, just reading this last sentence may still give you the chills!)

And if you're a woman, this may have been reinforced by the slow-dying social myth that "girls are innately not good at math." Unlearning any disabling anxiety is not a matter of suppressing or denying the phobia. It's more constructive to own your anxiety, to not be self-critical, and to take steps to overcome it. Here are three approaches to overcoming math anxiety.

First, realize that most business math is pretty simple. Sure, calculus and higher-order statistics are used in large corporate settings. But the basic arithmetic you studied in grammar school is all that is needed to understand and solve most practice-based business problems.

There are actually only two species of numbers for you to master, and both are pretty easy.

One set of numbers is "primary"—the number of patient visits seen in the clinic, for example, or the month-by-month collections. The other set of numbers are "derivatives." Most practice benchmarks fall into this category. Examples include the following:

- The average ticket (monthly collections divided by monthly patient visits)
- Surgical density (monthly visits divided by monthly surgical cases)
- Tech efficiency (monthly tech payroll hours divided by monthly visits)

As you can see, there's nothing more complex here mathematically than simple longhand division. You probably could have done these kinds of math problems when you were about 10 years old.

The biggest boost to understanding business math may not come from deciphering rows of abstract figures but from turning numbers into pictures. Take a glance at these two formats for looking at practice profits. Which is more readily understandable? The one on the left, or the one on the right?

	Annual Profit
2011	250,000
2012	243,000
2013	315,000
2014	375,000
2015	485,000
2016	695,000
2017	625,000
2018	600,000

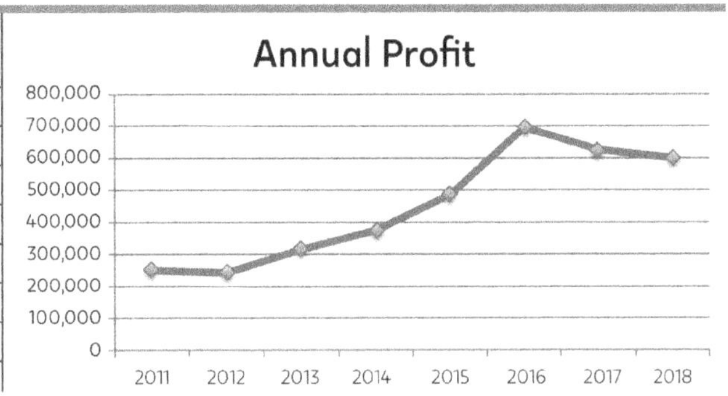

Second, talk to your employing physician. Odds are they had to be pretty good at math to have made it through training. Most of the eye surgeons I know enjoy teaching when approached the right way, and there's a hidden bonus: The kind of business math you need to master as an administrator is probably not all that familiar to your doctor, either. Make better business numeracy a challenge you work on together.

Last, harness your practice's accounting and consulting resources. Ask them to teach you how to read the monthly financial statements and how to calculate the most relevant benchmarks each quarter. Realize that just as your doctors turn to outside specialists at the local university to help them solve tough clinical cases, it's perfectly okay for you to turn to outside advisors when you're stumped with an unaccustomed round of business analysis.

• • •

As Beilock and her colleagues discovered, "It's not that math itself hurts. Rather, merely the anticipation of math is painful." So, the conclusion is clear if you are math phobic: Face up to the anxiety, fear, and pain that you associate with math—just start your computations. Face your fear and the pain will actually subside.

Of Measuring Efficiency

If you are the administrator of your practice, the first line of your job description would reasonably read: "Resource Allocation Authority." What resources do you have at your command to serve your patients and practice owners?

- Providers
- Lay staff

- Clinical and surgical facilities
- Technology
- Reputation
- Relationships
- Internal and external expertise
- And finally ... time

In years past, you could leave a lot of your potential resources lying fallow, because profit margins were so high. A generation ago, when one could easily bring 50% to the bottom line in an anterior segment practice, few really cared if there was an extra staffer up at the front desk, or if we ordered so many extra medical supplies that some of them went out of date before they could be used.

In the present and soon-to-come environment, that all changes. You not only need to think coarsely in terms of "Do we have any extra workers we don't really need?" but more granularly, "Can I send Mary home an hour early and bring $17 to the bottom line?"

As a practice manager, you may relish this new granular accountability. Indeed, if you came from tighter sectors of the economy—retail, restaurants, or hospitality—you're probably saying, "What took ophthalmology so long to catch up?"

You may already be benchmarking a few key indicators. Perhaps you have a formal dashboard of statistics you share with your board every month or quarter. Here's a possible augmentation to the benchmarking you already perform—a gross composite core of what percentage of your key resources you are actually using. This is a simple, fast way to objectively answer the question, "Are we doing all that we ***can*** with all that we ***have***?"

There are just three segments to this composite Ophthalmic Resources Utilization Score, or ORUS. Taken together, these three segments are not only the most important—they are also the most costly, consuming the aggregate of 70% or more of every dollar you collect. All three of these segments are couched in terms of what percentage of the maximum patient throughput each is achieving.

Provider Utilization Segment

All ophthalmologists and optometrists have their own personal capacity to see patients. I have MD clients who personally see more than 1000 visits per month. And others who groan at any more than 350 visits. How many patients you can see depends on a number of factors, but can be reduced to the following simple formulary:

- A general/geriatric or corneal ophthalmic provider is at 100% of nominal capacity at 550 visits (including postoperative, not including surgery or tech-only visits) per month.
- A plastics, retinal, glaucoma, or pediatric MD provider is at 100% at 450 visits per month.
- An optometrist, in the typical mid-level provider role, can comfortably see 350 visits per month.

Let's say your practice has one general ophthalmologist, one retinal specialist, and two ODs, named Smith, Jones, Davis, and Edwards, respectively. We'll call it Smith & Jones Eye. Make a table like the following:

Doctor	Average Monthly Patient Visits	Maximum Potential Monthly Patient Visits
Smith	500	550
Jones	375	450
Davis	450	350
Edwards	275	350
Total	**1600**	**1700**

Next, you can simply calculate what percent of nominal capacity your providers are at as a cohort by dividing their actual volume (1600) by their potential volume (1700), to get 94%.

Lay Staff Utilization Segment

Let's get to the second of three ORUS segments. There are several ways to measure lay staff efficiency. These include the following:

- Overall lay staff payroll hours per patient visit
- Tech, reception, or billing staff per visit transaction
- Staffing costs as a percent of collections
- Annual collections per full-time equivalent staffer in the practice

For the purpose of this ORUS system, we'll use a quite-close proxy for overall lay staffing efficiency—the number of "person-hours" per patient visit. You can calculate this very simply. Determine the average monthly core lay staff payroll hours the practice pays for—this can be readily determined from most payroll report forms. Omit surgical, optical, and contact lens staff. Divide the resulting hours by the average monthly patient visits in your practice.

In eye care, the high-water mark for this metric is 3.0 lay staff hours per patient visit—any higher and you are drowning in staff. A reasonable target in all segments except retina is 2.3 hours. In a pure retina practice, 2.6 hours is reasonable. In a hybrid practice, perhaps 2.5 hours. (It's interesting to know that it takes Toyota about 30 person-hours to build a car.)

So, let's imagine our sample practice (the one with four providers and 1600 visits per month) has 4480 lay staff payroll hours per month—that would be nearly 26 staffers. How do we calculate their efficiency score for this segment? Simple. First divide 4480 lay staff hours by 1600 visits, to get 2.8 staff hours per visit. Then (realizing that this is a mixed general-retinal practice and should have about 2.5 staff hours per visit) make the following calculation to get the efficiency percentage:

- With 4480 staff hours, they should be able to see 1792 patients per month (4480/2.5 = 1792).
- But, they actually only see 1600 visits.
- So, we divide 1600 by 1792 and get an efficiency percent of 89%.

Facility Utilization Segment

Last, we calculate facility utilization. How should that be done? Again, we resort to indexing to patient visits—this time, the relationship between exam rooms and examinations.

In the typical general practice, it takes one room hour to transit a patient visit. A practice like the one we are holding up as an example, with 1600 visits per month, requires 9.2 exam rooms (1600 visits divided by 173 hours in the average month).

But imagine that Smith & Jones Eye actually has 12 exam rooms. How many room hours do they have? And how do we calculate their utilization rate? Simple: 12 exam rooms times 173 hours in the average month makes for 2076 room hours. And they really only need 1600 room hours. So, we divide 1600 by 2076 and get 77%. (Note: There is not enough facility utilization difference between general practices and subspecialty practices to worry about—we simply use the metric of one exam room hour being needed per visit.)

• • •

The composite score in this example of Smith & Jones Eye is the average of the utilization scores:

(94% + 89% + 77%) / 3 = 87%

Said another way, Smith & Jones Eye is working at about 87% of its overall potential capacity. At what level should they be? That's entirely up to Smith & Jones, of course. But speaking economically, practice profitability improves the closer you can get to 100%.

Try this ORUS out in your own practice. If your score is lower than you would like, you have two options to improve: (1) to shed the excessive, expensive capacity or (2) to boost patient visits.

Of Growth, Stasis, and Shrinkage

Should we downsize, stay on the current plateau, or grow larger? At every size and stage every thoughtful practice owner asks several questions. How much larger should we grow? What risks am I willing to take? Will the rewards of growth be proportional or better to the hard work and sacrifice?

The correct answers to these questions can only emerge from an intersection between individual preferences, collective agreement in a multiowner practice, the available leadership resources, the limits imposed by your individual market environment, and what may be thought of as the "natural economic laws" of the business of eye care.

This is a highly nuanced area, with a large component relegated to the "feelings" category. You can't plug a few facts into your laptop and expect to have the best large, or small, answer emerge. The best growth game plan in the world is not going to be executed effectively unless the stakeholders are aligned and emotionally invested in the outcomes. This is why outside advisors may not be able to guide your practice's growth trajectory as well as you can, yourself, given a bit of quiet reflection and a candid discussion among the partners over where your priorities and values lie.

Beyond time and reflection, experience shows that leadership is the key resource for effective growth management. If you are stuck in your strategic planning, ask first, "Do we have a trusted, admired, energetic leader urging us forward?" Until you have at least one such individual, you're just going to be wandering randomly as a company, growing by opportunity, perhaps, but not by plan.

This is key. Even the largest practices typically grow larger not through the unified consensus of disparate owners, but with the unwavering, energetic urgings of a single physician-owner who enjoys the trust and admiration of the group. This leader is a foregone conclusion in a solo practice; it's much tougher in groups to pick someone. But whether the leader of your group practice is the oldest, the highest producer, or the doctor with the most free time, a leader is an essential precursor to planned, successful growth.

Growth from big to bigger, when you are in the middle of it, rarely feels consistently like it was a good idea. Taking on new doctors, services, and offices generally results in transient drops in profitability, and awkward lapses in customer service. The more growth investments you pack into a given year, the more that odds increase of a sharp drop in profit, operational fitness, or both. The faster you choose to grow, and the more risks you take, the more your trusted, admired, energetic leader has to give everyone the confidence needed to stay the course—much less change course and move in a new direction if you're on the wrong path.

To overcome this natural business rollercoaster, practices need several additional resources beyond great leadership, such as the following:

- True physician engagement, rather than the usual "presenteeism" evidenced on most doctor boards
- Partners who are managing their personal affairs to be able to live every month on far less than what they make, so that normal, transient business reversals are not so scary
- A strong practice administrator supported by deeply skilled middle managers
- The sense of control that comes with ever-improving daily operations
- A general momentum indicating success, despite occasional failure
- Capital reserves to overcome periodic reversals
- The judgment and confidence to change plans when conditions change

Every practice-owning surgeon has different ways of measuring whether efforts to grow are a success or a failure. Absolute financial measures are the core metric. Ask yourself, are we making more each year as we grow? But this is a very shallow measure. You have to look more deeply. In many practices I visit, partners in a growing organization will complain that their incomes have flattened or fallen.

Sometimes this is due to macroeconomic issues over which the practice has little control—fee reductions or local wage inflation. But more commonly, flat or falling partner income is due to a reduction in work hours and patient visits. It can be very helpful to measure each partner's net average profit per hour worked over time. A partner with no change in annual salary who has shifted from 5 days to 4 days of work per week, has actually enjoyed a material hourly pay raise.

For wise practices, successful growth is not measured in financial terms alone. There can be security and strategy rewards flowing from better contract access or larger community influence. There can be professional/intellectual rewards, working among a more diverse team of subspecialists. And, not to be overlooked, there can be ego rewards from a growing market share and even a measure of national prominence.

Unlike a publicly owned company, where "enhancing shareholder value" is by definition the highest goal, these metrics are personally and individually prioritized in a private ophthalmology practice.

How Big Is Too Big?

Most growing practices hit a developmental wall at around 8 to 12 surgeons, or about $10 million or so in annual net collections. Although there are mild economies of scale that attend growth—more intense equipment, staff, and facility use; better pricing for supplies; a degree of leveraged marketing—there can be even greater diseconomies of scale. These are largely driven by the logarithmic rise in complexity and doctor-to-doctor conflicts that bubble up to the surface as a practice grows. As a result, profit margins tend to peak in practice with about $8 million to $10 million in annual collections and then dip somewhat until a much, much larger scale is achieved.

There are only three possible responses to this well-documented difficulty seen as groups grow larger:

1. The group can revert back to a smaller scale where it's easier to achieve consensus, develop and execute a strategic plan, and preserve shareholder harmony.
2. The owners can plow ahead with modest levels of practice growth, and live with the resulting operational frustrations and mild to moderate diseconomies of scale—continuing to ask, often in vain, "Where are we going?" This is the most common state of affairs for larger practices.
3. The group can work hard and consciously to manifest the harmony, goal alignment, and leadership needed to derive an intelligent and inspirational growth plan and armor the owners for any necessary sacrifice, hard work, risk tolerance, and delayed gratification the plan may require. Such manifestation is the exception rather than the rule in eye care today.

How Is Medicine Different?

Ophthalmology is not an orthodox service business. In most service businesses—a chain of restaurants, let's say—the capitalist entrepreneur takes a predictable pathway. They invent a new service delivery model ... a new kind of restaurant in this case. They outlay the needed capital and open one outlet, often at great personal risk. This trial outlet is operated long enough to prove the business model and is polished along the way.

The food service entrepreneur then gets secondary financing to open additional outlets, each of which can eventually stand on its own without the daily attention of the founding owner because a growing management team is in place. There are subsequent rounds of growth, financing, and service improvement.

If successful, the owner can readily find a buyer—a private equity firm—or hit the jackpot of going public. If the owner is young, they can readily start all over again at the beginning and invent a new concept, this time with a much larger personal capital base.

This pathway is rarely followed by ophthalmic entrepreneurs for numerous reasons:

- Eye surgeons by their nature are much more risk averse than the average business entrepreneur. (This is paradoxical, of course—when an eye surgeon's business fails, they can typically secure a six-figure job offer in a few weeks.)
- Eye surgeons are raised up in a culture of perfection. Inasmuch as growth necessarily begets imperfection, growth can be restrained because "we're not perfect yet."
- Restaurants need managers, chefs, wait staff, and bookkeepers—all of whom are readily available at modest cost on the open market. Practices need surgeons, specialist-managers, experienced techs, billing and coding experts, etc.
- Restaurants have a relatively low level of enterprise complexity: a few dozen products, modest regulatory oversight, at-will pricing, simple accounting systems. Practices have a profoundly high level of enterprise complexity and regulatory oversight at all levels.
- With the right manager and chef, a restaurant owner can drop back from daily involvement and still collect a paycheck. It's far more difficult for an ophthalmologist-owner to run their practice passively—most qualified fellow surgeons are unwilling to generate passive incomes for owner-employers beyond a brief partner-track associate period.
- Practice succession is harder and less leveraged than ordinary business succession. Successful restaurant chains have a ready buyer pool who pay multiples of annual earnings. Ophthalmic practices sell today for their net tangible asset value plus a modest goodwill value … and the latter is slowly eroding.
- The new restaurateur can hold onto the dream that they will have a winning franchise concept and go public one day, netting tens or hundreds of millions of dollars. Few eye surgeons harbor such dreams.
- When a restaurant chain gets larger, its variable costs for food (which are high as a percentage of revenue) come down in percentile terms. In ophthalmology, most costs are fixed, not variable, so economies of scale are difficult to achieve.
- Most practices secure a customer base through the consistent excellence of their celebrity doctors; the ***doctor*** is the product. Restaurant chains secure a customer base by serving consistently great food; the ***food*** is the product. And with thousands upon thousands of new chefs graduating from culinary school every year,

the product is as much dependent on the recipe as on the maestro in an apron. You do not walk into an Applebee's and ask the hostess, "Who's in the kitchen tonight?"

That having been said, there are many motivations for buoyant practice growth to a larger scale:

- Theoretically, it will bring better access to contracts in the future.
- A large cohort of owners makes the buyout of any one owner easier.
- With more owners, the odds increase that at least one person will be willing and able to lead.
- With more owners, decisions are slower, but can be more rational. Rash, outlier opinions are dampened by a thoughtful majority.
- Large practices have the capital base to venture into riskier opportunities to drive passive income (eg, optical shops, ASCs, employed optometrists).
- The practice is less susceptible to the loss of any one key provider.
- The practice can afford a stronger management team, including in-house IT, marketing, and other specialists.
- There can be marketing economies of scale (ie, a $10 million practice would have to spend 9% of cash flow to have the same visibility in the market of a $30 million practice spending just 3%).
- There can also be modest optical, medical supply, and technology economies of scale.
- It makes possible coverage of a wider span of professional services and duplicate coverage for critical subspecialty areas.
- You'd have the pride of saying, "We are the largest practice in the area."

To balance out this list of growth drivers, there are nearly as many motivations for relative stasis or even downsizing your practice from where it stands today. There are well-recognized difficulties seen with large-scale practices, both economically and interpersonally. There is better proportionality between practice scale and doctor leadership resources; there are low odds of finding an engaged partner with free time to be the serious executive needed in a large practice.

With fewer owners, decisions are faster. Both large and small practices have ready access to money for worthy business ideas in today's capital markets, so you do not need to get bigger to fund new projects. Importantly, practice problems are largely caused by people. Odds are that a practice with twice the number of doctors, staff, and patients will have at least twice the problems of smaller practices. Ted Turner, of CNN and bison ranching fame, once quipped, "Problems are equal to the number of people … squared."

Finally, most eye surgeons are pretty individualistic, control-oriented people. Bankers and sales executives and lawyers who used to play football may inherently love being part of a large corporate team. But as a general observation, ophthalmologists tend to be happy in their businesses in inverse proportion to practice size.

Half the calls I get for help are from large and growing practices, and the other half are from smaller practices working to stay that way and remain profitable. With any luck, there will be a place for both business models long into the future.

Of the Three Buckets of Money

With advance apologies, let's be crass and discuss an odd taboo of American ophthalmic culture, your personal income. Money. Cash. Dough. Wealth. Moolah.

If you are a surgeon reading this, chances are slim that you have pointed to a figure on a page and told your administrator and your colleague-doctors, point blank, "Here is the income I would like to earn this year." Chances are equally low that your OM, administrator, or even your accountant have asked you about a finite income target. Even if they did ask, you would be more likely to say, "More," than to declare a definitive goal.

And yet, this is the bottom line metric for every discussion you ***should*** be having with your partners and managers.

I'd like to help you break through the taboo of declaring what you really want to make, and free you up for some essential, if sometimes uncomfortable, confrontations about money.

The Three Buckets of Money

Let's say your practice will be throwing off half a million dollars in available profit after all expenses this year. What can you spend? What should you save?

There are only three fundamental "buckets" into which you could be spilling these profits:

1. *Reinvestments back into the business*—funds you use to purchase new capital equipment, bet on a new office satellite, or use to bankroll a partner-track associate
2. *Future lifestyle dollars*—the income you save for retirement, largely in tax-favored pension plans
3. *Current lifestyle dollars*—the income you bring home, pay taxes on, and use to pay the mortgage, the grocery bills, and your child's English riding lessons

The order in which you fund each of these buckets, and the discipline with which you do so, is critical. Deciding how much to put into each bucket is at the core of every decision you make in the boardroom, whether yours is a solo practice or a group, and whether you are nearing retirement or still decades away from winding down your career.

Filling Practice Needs First

The first priority—the first bucket—should be your practice. Starving the proverbial golden goose of needed resources will result in an eventual downward profit spiral. A common observation today, as fees are falling and expenses rising, is for owners to draw accustomed amounts from their practices, leaving behind deferred maintenance, unrewarded staff, and marketing underinvestment. A few cycles of this parsimony can materially reduce your practice's ability to rise to the next business opportunity, much less recover from the next business shock or competitive threat.

An excellent discipline to adopt from the outset of a young, new practice is to set aside a reserve fund of about 10% of practice earnings—more if you have high ambitions—for future investment.

Let's look at why this disciplined reserve fund is important. Say you launch a solo practice and 8 years later decide to add a partner-track associate. In today's tight labor market, the cost of recruiting and carrying a new associate for the first year or so of practice will be a minimum of $200,000. This cost would be painless if you had built up a war chest of practice development funds—but very difficult to contemplate if you had been drawing and living on 100% of available profits from the practice each year.

Even if you can't quite yet imagine what you would use the funds for, start saving at least 10% of your available cash flow today for future development.

Future Lifestyle Savings

The second bucket of money you should fill is your retirement fund. Ideally, yours is not the average American family that today, incredibly, spends nearly everything it makes and saves little for retirement. Instead, applying somewhat more prudence than that, you should plan when you reach full retirement to have invested funds under management equal to about 25 times your expected annual lifestyle costs. Make that 30 times if you are more conservative.

To enjoy a $100,000 retirement lifestyle, you should retire with not less than $2.5 million in appropriately invested assets.

Depending on how early or late you plan to retire, and on how conservatively or aggressively you invest your retirement savings, it's essential to be setting aside 10% to 20% of available profits for retirement—***before*** you start spending the rest on current lifestyle costs.

Current Lifestyle Needs and Wants

The last bucket of money can be drawn out to pay current lifestyle costs, including taxes, mortgages and loans, vacations, food, clothing, shelter, school fees, entertainment, ***and*** those inevitable riding lessons.

• • •

The Question Managers Should Ask Their Doctors

This is all leading up to one seminal question that every manager should ask each of the practice's doctors annually: "How much do you need to make this year?" Based on the previous conservative approach, the following simple math steps would apply to an imaginary Dr. Jenny Jones:

- The doctor and her family determine that Dr. Jones needs to cover personal lifestyle costs of $300,000 per year.
- Remembering that such costs should consume not more than about 75% of available profits from the practice (leaving aside, let's say, 15% for retirement savings and a 10% reserve of profit for investments back in for practice growth), this means that Dr. Jones needs to generate profits of $400,000.
- In the typical very well-run practice today, with profit margins of about 40%, it takes net collections of $1 million to leave behind $400,000 in free cash flow available to fund buckets 1, 2, and 3.

Let's imagine that Dr. Jones is only generating about $900,000 in annual collections at present. And let's say she does so by seeing about 484 patients per month, with an average revenue yield of $155 per visit. Something has to change to net out at $300,000 for current lifestyle costs, right? Yes, and there are at least five options for Dr. Jones to consider—several dependent variables she can adjust singly or in combination:

1. She could work a bit harder and see roughly 538 patients per month—or a bit more than three more patients per day in a 4-day clinic week, 48 weeks per year, compared to today.
2. She could become more aggressive with testing and surgery, and boost the average revenue yield per patient visit to about $173.
3. She could invest more aggressively, and hope that higher returns on her retirement funds will make up for setting aside lower dollar amounts each year.
4. She could retire a few years later than planned, reducing the cushion of funds needed for retirement.
5. She could reduce current as well as postretirement lifestyle costs, creating a lower demand for ramping up clinical production.

Obviously, all of these gross example figures for Dr. Jones are going to be impacted by at least two other variables that she will have essentially zero control over: the pace of inflation and the rate at which third-party fees are reduced in the years ahead. However, by adjusting those variables and dimensions that are under her control, Dr. Jones can pursue a more deliberate, intentional career and achieve a much deeper working relationship with her partners and administrative staff.

If you decide to apply this logical set of calculations to your own situation, be sure to bring the resulting estimates home to share with your spouse, because most of the production or budget adjustments that you'll likely need to make—working harder, working differently, or spending less—may have a direct impact on your family life.

By working backward in a very simple fashion, from an approximation of your current or desired lifestyle costs, you can achieve greater control over the path ahead and have much greater certainty that the strategic course of your practice is congruent with your interests and the needs of every practice stakeholder.

Of Objectifying That Which Is Subjective

In 1900, Lord William Thomson Kelvin, the great Scottish mathematician and physicist, addressed the British Association for the Advancement of Science and stated, "There is nothing new to be discovered in physics. All that remains is more and more precise measurement."

Lord Kelvin also said, "When you can measure what you are talking about and express it in numbers, you know something about it."

He was as spectacularly wrong on the first count, as he was spot on in his observation that measurement begets understanding. This applies as much in high-level physics today as it does in your progressively more difficult labors to run an efficient, effective ophthalmic practice-business.

Much in the business of medicine is perfectly calculable. With your practice management system and a few million keystrokes a year you can track service counts, patient visits, collections, no-shows, denial rates, and scores of derivative benchmarks like the average collections yielded by a single visit, your practice's comparative surgical density, and your surgeon's assertiveness in special testing. With the latest electronic medical records, you can perform regression analysis on the impact of various treatments and surgical approaches in your hands.

Meanwhile, your bookkeeper and accountant should be able to generate and interpret all the key performance indicators signaling your practice's business health: profit margins, various cost ratios, capital reserves, and the like.

But there is another class of analytics available, something you are very familiar with as a physician, but are probably not using as a business owner or manager. It is the kind of analysis that comes from turning something that is essentially subjective into something objective and comparable on a relative scale.

Here is an example. There is not a lot of pain treatment associated with ophthalmology, but from your training days you'll recall how internists and nurses commonly ask their patients, "On a 1 to 10 scale, where 1 is low and 10 is high, what is your current level of pain?"

This is a brilliant question that helps to get around the fact that an electronic "pain-o-meter" does not yet exist. So, physicians and nurses have to resort to asking their patients how they feel. But rather than asking a question that will yield a mushy answer like "It hurts a lot," doctors ask in a way that gives a progressive score. One patient's "9" may be another's "6", but asking for a ***number***—especially over time—communicates relative treatment progress, healing, expectations, and accountability.

Let's apply this familiar and useful medical contrivance to the business side of your practice in three different dimensions.

Staff Performance

More than 3 decades ago when I started in this business, I'd ask a doctor client, "What's your impression of your staff?" That simple question would often lead to hours of narrative, peppered with words like "dreadful" or "spectacular" or "overworked."

Later, I learned a simple expedient to help doctors get to the point faster and more clearly. I'd simply ask three focused questions about each staff member:

1. What's Norah's current global performance score on a 1 to 10 scale (like a patient's pain score, right?)—including everything: timeliness, coworker relations, job knowledge, customer service, and the rest?
2. What's Norah's potential score?
3. What would Norah need to do to reach this potential score?

The result in your setting may look something like this:

Staffer/ Position	Current Global Performance Score (1=low, 10=high)	Potential Score	Notes and Next Action
Norah/ Head Tech	7	9	Norah has been distracted this year by petty conflicts between staff members on the floor. Bring in an outside trainer to work with the entire team and to provide focused leadership coaching for Norah. Remove Amy, who is "stirring the pot" and resisting Norah's role as her manager. Annex Dr. Arnold to the tech team for the next year to help with continuing education sessions and to back Norah up publicly. Set a deadline for writing the new tech training manual.
Frank/ Optician	4	5	After 2 years on staff, it is clear that Frank is not going to reach the sales levels we expect of our dispensing opticians. Replace in the next 120 days.
Mary/ Billing Clerk	9	9+	We could not function without Mary on the team. She generates much more than her fair share of the billing work, and does so cheerfully, even when one of her two billing colleagues is out of the office for a week. Although she does not yet possess the maturity to lead the department, she should be advanced formally as the understudy for Susan, who will be retiring in 18 months.

Vendor Performance

The same 1 to 10 scale can be used to perform an annual evaluation for the key vendors serving your practice. Make up a grid like the one below and enter your principle outside vendors in the first column. In the second column, write down their global score ... Is pricing fair? ... Is the service timely? ... Do they follow through on their promises? In the last column, write down the next action you're going to take.

Just as vision comes in plus, minus, and plano, your vendors probably fall into similar categories: vendors you want to hold onto forever, vendors you need to improve soon or terminate, and vendors between these two extremes.

When you make up a grid like this, it may look something like this:

Vendor	Global Score (1 to 10)	Next Action
Jones Plumbing & Heating	4... on our last service call, their technician took 5 hours to solve a simple problem, and they tried to charge us for 6 hours	Try Smith Plumbing at the time of the next service call and, if satisfactory, negotiate a 10% hourly fee discount to be our regular vendor
Ruth's Cleaning Service	9... consistently exceeds our expectations	Letter of thanks from the board, and a small holiday gift

Rating Your Current Computer System

When I ask frontline ophthalmic workers what they think of their current practice management or EHR system, they respond in several ways. Some respond nonverbally with a sour face, or a wide smile and a thumbs-up. Others, especially those who are detail-oriented, will go on for several minutes outlining selected strong and weak points, but no overall rating.

As a consultant, neither of these responses are terribly useful. So, a long time ago I started asking in a different way:

- If your computer system was a student, and you were the teacher, what letter grade (eg, A-, B+) would you give it?
- What would your current system vendor need to do differently to deserve a higher grade?
- What's the minimum acceptable grade an IT system must earn in this practice to remain and not be replaced by something better?

• • •

Questions like this—questions that make the responder rate systems and commit to a specific, narrow score—are part of the simple, inner game of ophthalmology. Whether you pose these objective questions to yourself when thinking about your company or use them to stimulate a group discussion, communication will improve, staff reports will be more precise, and your people will be more accountable for agreed outcomes. Be a follower of René Descartes, the great 17th-century French mathematician who said, "With me everything turns into mathematics."

Of Benchmarking

A standard or point of reference against which things may be compared or assessed.
—The Oxford English Dictionary

Pity the poor Renaissance physician. There was but one lab test in prominent use at the time: to examine and then ***taste*** a sick patient's urine. With professional rigors such as this, I'm sure there were very few complaints back then from doctors like the ones heard today—about falling fees or weekend call duty.

Four centuries later, clinical analysis became more fastidious and reproducible. In 1896 the first US clinical laboratory was opened at a cost of $50 at Johns Hopkins Hospital. Modern, fact-based medicine was born. It thrives now, with thousands of assays, tests, and associated "within normal limits" (WNLs) to memorize in medical school.

Of course, for ophthalmologists at least, there are no more than 100 or so of these clinical norms to fuss with on an average day. Aside from the occasional interesting case, you only have to worry about WNLs for visual acuity and intraocular pressure, field of vision, cup-to-disc ratio, and the like.

Every ophthalmologist reading this book could give an impromptu 20-minute lecture on the most recent patient they saw in clinic. Many could do so without notes in front of them. With a chart open, every eye surgeon I've ever met could stand and deliver at length with facts and figures galore.

I bring this up to illustrate the comparatively more primitive state of ophthalmic business management today. It is only in the last generation that robust financial analysis and benchmarking have been introduced in eye care, and only in the last few years has some of this finally trickled down to the average practice.

Consider the contrast. While every ophthalmologist could impressively sum up a patient's eye health status, far fewer than half of the surgeons reading this have administrators who could perform the business equivalent. And these administrators only have *one* patient—your practice.

Indeed, in about one out of every five practices that I come across, the OM isn't even granted access to the financial reports of the practice—the business cognate of the "lab report." That would be like you walking into the next exam room and saying, "Nice blue eyes, Mildred. Looks good to me. See you in a year."

Do not run out and put your manager on the spot—at least not yet, but consider what your administrator could do for your business if they were as strong at the technical aspects of caring for your practice as you are at taking care of your patients, and could rattle off something like:

> Jones Eye Associates is a 45-year-old general ophthalmology and optometry practice. Our primary service area is Smith, Davis, and Westfield Counties, which have a combined drawing area of 253,000 people and a population-to-provider ratio of 32,000. This makes our area comparatively underserved. We are ranked number two in local market share behind Higgins Eye Institute, and enjoy 23% of the global area eye care market and 55% of the local cataract care. For the first two quarters of

> this year, practice net revenue is up 8% over the same period last year, indicating that we are gaining relative market share. We are currently on track to hit 42% consolidated cash-basis profit margins, with the average partner taking home about 53% of their personal collections, if current trends hold. This favorable profit margin is driven by three core factors. First, we have a surgically dense practice with only eight visits per surgical case. This, in turn, gives us higher collections per patient visit—$198 compared to averages of $160 in fellow practices. Second, we have a much higher level of labor productivity than peer practices, with just 2.1 lay staff hours per patient visit. Finally, we locked in a very low price on office facilities 6 years ago, and with subsequent growth, facility costs are now running only 4% of cash flow. The most important opportunity we have coming up next is the development of a surgery center, which will provide an extra $290 in income per cataract case, and over the next 10 years will boost our average partner's net worth by about $1.3 million.

Chances are that your administrator is not ***quite*** there yet. But they could be very soon with your encouragement.

Just as physicians became more effective through the centuries by objectifying symptoms and signs and codifying the best treatment approaches, so too could your administrator become more effective. And it won't take centuries, because most of the work has already been done. The foundation for administrative improvement is benchmarking.

Here is a starter kit of 20 important benchmarks to master:

1. *Net revenue growth rate.* If you ever watch corporate CEOs being interviewed about their company's performance, one core statistic they refer to often is "sales," which in ambulatory health care settings is more genteelly called "collections," "revenue," or "net revenue." Practice revenue growth rate is simply the collections this year, minus collections for the prior year, divided by the collections for the prior year. For example, a practice that collected $1 million last year and $1.1 million this year enjoyed a 10% growth rate. What should your practice's revenue growth rate be? Inasmuch as the demand for ophthalmic services is growing at roughly 4% per year, that would be a reasonable baseline goal. At a 4% growth rate you'll neither lose nor gain market share, and you'll be able to keep your head above general practice cost inflation. Young and aggressive practices should aim at 10% growth rates; mature practitioners gliding toward retirement can do just fine with zero net revenue growth, or even a slow decline if there is no plan to pass the practice on to a successor.
2. *Profit and cost margins.* Your practice's profit, by industry convention, includes all MD or DO salaries, taxes, benefits, and dividends. To get the profit margin, simply divide this profit number by total collections. A practice with $1 million in net collections, and with $350,000 in salaries for the physicians, has a 35% profit margin and a 65% cost margin. Profit margin norms today range widely from 30% to 45% in suburban general practice. Urban practices with high operating costs and low managed care payments can be "normal" with a 25% or lower profit margin.

Rural general practices with low overhead and even lower levels of competition can hit 50% margins. Well-run retinal and plastics practices commonly achieve 50+% profit margins.

3. *Collections per average patient visit.* This benchmark is also commonly referred to as the "average ticket." This is another easy calculation to make. Take the total monthly collections and divide by monthly total patient visits (inclusive of postoperative visits). A typical figure for a general ophthalmologist is $150 or higher. You can expect another $25 or more if the practice dispenses glasses. Optometrists on your staff will probably have an average ticket of $125 or less. Surgically assertive practices, and practices with a high pathology mix (and lots of special testing), commonly hit $225 or more. Average ticket figures for retinal practices commonly hit $250 and up. (*Note:* Considering the convention in retinal practices with high drug costs, which are essentially a pass-through expense, one wants to omit from the collections figure any drug reimbursements.)
4. *Core cost per patient visit.* This benchmark provides a very useful practice-to-practice comparison, and is also a useful wake-up call for practices with runaway operating costs. Again, the math is easy. Add up total annual practice costs before all optical or contact lens goods costs; before depreciation; before all providers' wages, taxes, and/or benefits; and before any exceptional cost of sales, such as injectable drugs, premium IOLs, or LASIK center fees. Divide the resulting figure by the number of patient visits per year, including postoperative visits. If you have a highly efficient practice, your number will be at or under $90. If you have an average practice in America today, your figure may be closer to $120. But this figure is as unhealthy for your practice as a high body mass index is for your health. Lower is better.
5. *Staffing cost ratio.* The highest single cost category in virtually all practices is lay staffing. Simply divide total lay staff payroll, benefits, and taxes by total practice collections (again, net of drug reimbursements). The typical value in a well-run, suburban general ophthalmology practice today is 28% to 33%. Depending upon your practice type and setting, this ratio may be higher or lower in your practice. Retinal and plastics practices with higher revenue yields per patient visit commonly get by spending 25% or less. Urban surgeons with lower managed care payments and higher wage demands can expect 35% or higher costs without careful efforts at cost containment.
6. *Facilities cost ratio.* In most practices, the second largest cost after lay staffing is the cost of facilities. Simply add up the relevant annual costs—rent or principle/interest payments, utilities, taxes, and basic repairs—and divide by annual collections. In the typical setting, 4% to 6% is reasonable. The cost ranges to 10% or more if you practice in the high-priced urban core or have recently developed a new facility that your practice is still growing into. Fortunate rural providers often get by on a 2% or lower facilities cost and bring the extra percentage points to the bottom line of their practice.
7. *Marketing cost ratio.* The overall cost to generate new patients is commonly the third highest practice expense. This includes inexpensive elements like recall and customer service tune-ups, outreach to referral sources, and community eye

screenings—but also, in the most aggressive settings, includes direct-to-consumer advertising. Add up all your marketing, advertising, and PR costs and divide by practice collections. For the average, mid-career general ophthalmologist, 2% to 4% of cash flow spent on marketing communications is perfectly sufficient; spending less than this may cause your practice to atrophy. Costs rise to the 10% to 15% level in elective plastics or LASIK settings, especially in larger cities where competition is high and media costs can be astounding. Old-line, established practices with no further growth aspirations and referral-dependent retinal practices commonly get by on less than 2%.

8. *Patient visits per exam room hour.* Have you ever wondered how your practice compares to others in terms of the efficient use of office space? Here's how you can do it. Add up the total patient visits for the year (including postoperative) and divide by the number of exam room hours per year, which is calculated by taking the number of fully equipped exam rooms times the 2080 nominal potential hours available to see patients per year. The typical figure is ± 1.0 patient visit per exam room per hour, a figure that generally holds up whether the practice is performing general or subspecialty care. If the figure you get in your practice is 0.7, that means you're only using about 70% of your available facilities. If the number comes out significantly higher than 1.0 (let's say 1.2 or 1.4), you are probably overwhelming your current physical plant. Options include expanding hours, shedding lower-paying or less professionally interesting categories of patients, or adding more exam rooms and collateral space.
9. *Information technology cost ratio.* A couple of decades ago, the IT costs in your practice were scant in relation to annual collections. The typical practice management systems and their upkeep only cost about 2% or less of cash flow. Any mid-level OM could readily handle the duties of key operator—you didn't need much of a technical services team on call. Not so today. EHRs and related consulting and support services have plumped up the cost to $25,000 or more per doctor per year. Add up all your annual preventative maintenance (PM)/EHR software, support, hardware, consulting, web access, and related costs and divide by collections. You may be shocked to see a cost that was once under 2% is now hitting as much as 5% of your cash flow.
10. *Technician efficiency ratio.* To derive this figure, add up all tech payroll hours in an average month (including work-up techs, scribes, and testing staff) and divide by the number of patient visits, inclusive of postoperative visits. This figure was once as low as 0.6 or 0.7 tech hours per visit in a general ophthalmology practice, but now stands at 0.9 to 1.0 with the advent of more available testing. Retinal practices benchmark at 1.3 and pure LASIK practices at about 1.1 tech hours per visit. The figure can be somewhat higher in a practice that delegates more care to lay staff, or a practice with lots of trainees, or a hub-and-spoke practice with lots of time lost to travel.
11. *Reception staff efficiency ratio.* This includes all check-in and check-out staff, anyone answering the phones or making appointments, and anyone trafficking medical records. Be sure to omit any time spent by these same staff posting charges (eg, some well-run practices post charges at the front desk at checkout). Take the staff

total payroll hours and divide by total patient visits, including postoperatives. The typical figure is now 0.4 to 0.5 in ophthalmic practices of any composition.

12. *Percent of total receivables.* Over 90 days. This figure is found in every practice management system's aging report, typically appearing on the last page of the printout. The figure we like to see is 12% or lower for the typical general/geriatric practice; half of this in a practice with a significant cash-and-carry trade (eg, elective plastics, LASIK, optical).
13. *Patient accounts staff efficiency.* Add up the billing department's total payroll hours (eg, all staff doing posting, charging, collections) and divide by the additive product of the total patient visits (inclusive of postoperatives) and the total surgical cases. The average figure seen is 0.3 staff hours per transaction. Astoundingly, in America today, it takes about 18 minutes of clerical time for you to get paid for each average patient service rendered. For comparison, my Canadian clients typically get the job done in 5 minutes or less.
14. *Surgical counselor efficiency.* With the advent of premium lens options, the role of the surgical counselor has expanded from mere clerking and patient hand-holding. The extra teaching and motivating time is better for the patient and certainly better for the practice. Add up surgical counseling staff hours per average month and divided by the number of surgical cases per average month. With 173 payroll hours in an average month, the typical full-time counselor can transit 50 to 150 cases per month—that comes to 1.2 to 3.5 payroll hours per case. The metric is wide-ranging based on staff experience, the premium IOL implant rate of the practice, your control over the surgical facilities used, and the scope of counselor responsibility.
15. *Patient visits per ophthalmic surgeon per month.* For general ophthalmology, the figure optimally lies at 550 visits or more, including postoperative care. In a subspecialist's practice, ± 450 is a reasonable target.
16. *Percent of allotted schedule template that is filled.* Trick question: If a doctor's half-day session allots 25 appointment slots, what percentage of these slots should actually be filled at the start of each day, before cancellations and no-shows? 100% is obviously the correct answer, but do not be surprised if the answer in your practice is well under 100%. A few empty appointment slots may sound like no big deal—even a nice respite—but just three missing patients per clinic day can skim more than $100,000 from your bottom line.
17. *No-show rates.* This is the percentage of today's scheduled patients, even after prior reminder calls have been placed, who did not show up today for their appointment. A clinic with 100 filled appointments when the day started, and four missing patients throughout the course of the day would have a 4% no-show rate. This figure should be averaged over longer time frames, by location, and by provider. A 5% or lower figure is desirable in a general practice. Rates commonly hit 7% to 15% in pediatric offices, optometric clinics, settings with a higher percentage of Medicaid patients, and in urban (as compared to rural) practices.
18. *Surgical density.* This benchmark, which is most applicable to a cataract practice but also germane in retinal settings, measures the number of patient visits (including postoperative) your practice transits per surgical case. The average seen today

is 25 visits per case (eg, a practice with 600 visits per month would typically transit about 24 surgical cases). This figure can range widely and is best used by each surgeon as a personal benchmark and reference standard, and a starting point for improvement. The figure is often well under 10 visits per case in an optometric co-management setting. A newly graduated surgeon may benchmark at 40 or 50 visits per case, in part due to an appropriately conservative approach to case selection.

19. *Annual lay staff separation rate.* This benchmark is a useful proxy for the job you are doing with new hires and with human resource management. It costs dearly to train and then lose a valued staff member. So, within bounds, we want to have the lowest possible separation rate. Divide the number of lay staff departures (voluntary and involuntary) you have experienced in the last 12 months by the average number of lay staff members who have been employed by your practice during the same period. Then multiply that number by 100 to express the benchmark as a percentage. The US private industry rate is about 37%. The figure is only around 15% in government service. In the typical, well-run ophthalmic practice, with good hiring and tenure-boosting policies, we typically see about 25%—that is to say, the average ophthalmic worker in America lasts on average about 4 years on the job before moving on.
20. *Profit per surgeon-hour.* This is a critical metric. Perhaps ***the*** critical measure of the sum-total of your practice's performance. Divide each physician's annual wages, taxes, and benefits by their number of professional hours (including administrative and meeting time). The figure can be wide ranging—it may be as little as $50 or well over $600. This is one of many dimensions of efficiency measurement where ratio analysis is best applied as an *internal* standard, rather than trying to match *external* benchmarks. Measure your current number and then, like a motivated runner, aim for a new "personal best."

How often should these basic benchmarks be tracked? Most of these statics do not change very much over a period of several quarters. Obviously, key stats like your practice's profit margin and labor cost should be examined in the monthly financial statements. Other statistics, derivatives like the average collections per patient visit, can be fascinating to track graphically over the last 2 or 3 years. And some data like facility costs are only useful when examined at longer intervals.

• • •

A final thought … in medicine, we only want to gather information that is going to be useful in making a clinical decision, right? No ophthalmology charts I've ever seen have a place to record a patient's favorite color, because this information has no bearing on patient care.

The same, simple logic applies in business. While many of the benchmarks covered in this book may be fascinating to look at one time, you need only track longitudinally those data that will help you and your management team make better business decisions.

Of Financial Sufficiency

What a funny term, "liquidity management." What does it mean? Does it refer to keeping saline on an intraoperative eye? Staying hydrated during your next 10K run? Stocking up adequately for this Friday night's party so the punchbowl doesn't run dry?

Nope. None of these, at least if you own or manage a practice-business.

Liquidity management is a core business discipline, and perhaps one of the most important skills you'll want to improve in the years ahead, as profit margins thin and the typical practice board member becomes inclined to take every last dollar of free cash flow out of the practice to sustain doctor lifestyles.

"Liquidity" is simply another term for financial sufficiency, your access to capital ... cash ... ***right*** now. If yours is a highly liquid practice, you have lots of cash or cash-equivalents at the ready. These equivalents can include the following:

- One or more lines of credit at your commercial bank
- The doctor's access to available personal funds
- Home equity credit lines that haven't been tapped
- The practice's accounts receivable, to the extent they might be used as collateral by a receivables factoring company in a pinch

Liquidity is ***not*** the value of your optical frames on the wall or your drug inventory. It's not the value of your office building (unless you could rapidly sell it and lease it back). And it's not future earnings, which are not available if you need access to a near-term infusion of cash.

Liquidity was once no big deal in the business of eye care.

Younger readers won't remember, but there was a time in this profession when cataract surgery paid nearly $5000 in terms of today's devalued currency, and profit margins were commonly above 50%. In this long-ago environment, even the most humble, under-earning ophthalmologist could live in the nicest house in town, drive off in the nicest car on the lot, and still sock away half of their salary to loan back to their practice on a rainy day.

It was also an era of lower risks: lower competition, fewer slip-and-fall lawsuits—along with cheaper risk management. It was once a snap to get a disability policy that could almost immediately replace all of your income.

No so much anymore. Liquidity is something that must now be closely managed. And you'll have to watch it like a hawk in the years ahead, when the economic ecology of eye care could be vastly different.

Here are some basic pointers to get you started:

1. Keep your eye on three key domains, all of which drive the need for your ready access to capital:
    - *Cash flow fluctuations.* As described previously, most practices have a soft first quarter. An increasing number even have 1 or 2 months each year (as is common for retailers and restaurateurs) where, as the old saying goes, "Your outgo exceeds your income, so your upkeep becomes your downfall." They run in the red.

- *Unplanned events.* Some things like fire, flood, and doctor disability can be insured against; other things cannot. What if you're in a two-doctor practice and your partner leaves? You'll have to buy them out. You will lose their revenue production (while covering the fixed costs they left behind). And you'll have the considerable cost and time delays of finding a new doctor to take their place. You can calmly get through a crisis like that if you have an extra half-million dollars at the ready.
- *Opportunities.* What if a nearby competitor retires abruptly and you can only win a bidding war for their practice if you can come up with cash? Or if you come across a terrific potential partner-track associate, but when they are hired, you're going to have a lean year personally covering their salary and costs until their practice develops? Think back. Every year there has probably been at least one great opportunity that you had to pass up because you didn't have enough of a cushion to be bold.

2. You need to know where you want to head. Look at the previous three domains … estimate what kind of cushion you need—add it up—and then throw in a little extra that will help you sleep at night. Here is an example, imagining a fairly prosperous two-doctor practice, Smith Eye:
   - *Fluctuations.* Smith Eye is in the snow belt. Both doctors like to take 1 month off in winter, which makes sense since many of their patients also fly south. They have 2 months, January and February, when core expenses are barely covered and doctor draws are lean. They review the numbers and see that the difference between a poor month and an average month is $50,000 in net cash flow. So, they need a revolving ***$100,000*** or so in the kitty to cover cash flow fluxes and the occasional blizzard.
   - *Unplanned events.* The two doctors who own Smith Eye enjoy practicing together so much that neither is going to leave voluntarily. And all the usual contingencies—death and disability, fire and flood, and the like—are more than adequately covered by insurance. All except for one biggie—a Medicare fee cut. The doctors figure that based on their current overhead structure, if there is a 10% fee cut (the most they imagine happening in any 1 year) they will have a net 15% pay cut. They think it will take the better part of a year to sort things out, reduce personal and practice costs, and boost patient volumes. They each make $350,000 a year now. A 15% pay cut on a $700,000 combined owner distribution comes to ***$105,000***.
   - *Opportunities.* The owners of Smith Eye are pretty conservative, and both are in their late 50s. They are not interested in buying up practices or getting new equipment—but they *are* going to be hiring a new partner-track doctor in about 1 year. They figure the new doctor will start covering their costs after the first year, but could end up being a net drain of ***$150,000*** in the first year, a bit more if things do not work out well.

- So, all up, Smith Eye probably wants to have not less than $355,000 in liquid, readily accessible funds; $400,000 would be better. They set this higher figure as their target.

3. *Bridge the gap.* If you own Smith Eye and need $400,000 in liquid funds on hand, and only have $200,000, you're $200,000 short. The doctors of Smith Eye could catch up in several ways. They could catch up slowly by withholding an affordable portion of their draws for a couple of years. They could swiftly catch up by taking out a new line of credit, or pledging a portion of their personal funds to the practice in the event of an emergency. They could even nibble away at the gap a bit by taking less vacation and improving their first-quarter operating performance. Or, they could catch up by delaying the admission of a new associate until the practice is so busy that the new provider is immediately productive as soon as they arrive.

• • •

There has never been a more critical time than now to start actively managing the liquidity of your practice. With a bit of planning, you can painlessly sequester capital— and capital access— that will help you sleep more soundly and manage your organization from a position of strength.

Of Staff Cost Containment

The following exercise will be the least expensive management lesson you get this week.

Assuming you are sitting down at your desk, put down this book for a minute, reach into your wallet or purse, and pull out a dollar bill. With a pair of scissors, cut away the left third of the bill—right about where the "T" is in the word "United." Put the larger part of the bill back in your wallet.

This one-third slice remaining represents the approximate fraction of every dollar your practice collects that goes back out to pay the wages, benefits, taxes, and related support costs for your lay staff. It is your number-one practice cost today. Therefore, it needs to be your number one focus for cost containment.

Now tape that one-third of a dollar somewhere you'll see it daily, and continue reading.

• • •

In the present environment of stagnant professional fees and humane limits on how much longer and more intensely you can work every day, your mandate (if you want to preserve personal income) is to shrink the size of that dollar clipping.

Here are 20 approaches to stabilizing and reducing labor costs. Some of these approaches may sound harsh. No doctor or administrator relishes taking hours or benefits away from workers. But the present business context has a clinical analog: Patients sometimes must accept unpleasant procedures to see better or stay alive. In this case, your practice (which may now be supporting dozens of families, including your own) is more important than any individual worker.

1. *Learn what your real labor needs are.* Industry norms have now been long established for how many staff you really need. Go back and read the section of this book on Benchmarking.
2. *Eliminate the 40-hour-week entitlement.* If you must, reduce average weekly payroll hours to those levels actually needed by the practice; wean staff from the expectation of a 40-hour work week. You wouldn't lease a 2000-square-foot office if you only needed 1500 square feet. Only pay for the labor you need, anything more is wasted.
3. *Know your local market's customary labor rates.* If you practice in rural America, do not read too much into national salary surveys. Survey neighboring practices and peg your wage scale to local norms.
4. *Realize that people work for love plus money.* If you are a beast to work for, you will have to bribe your most capable people to stick around. If you take your charm pills every morning, it will reduce the pace of wage inflation in your practice and you will see labor costs fall as a percent of collections.
5. *Change provider behaviors.* Be a bit more Yankee. Do it yourself when this is more cost-effective. I've seen providers who insist on two assistants in the room, one to scribe and one to instill drops and help a patient center their chin in the slit lamp. Unless you make rock-star wages, reduce your dependency on an entourage of support staff.
6. *As feasible, replace full-time workers with part-time staff.* You will save benefits costs and potentially increase the elasticity of your practice's capacity (eg, having a 28-hour worker come in additional hours to cover for a temporarily absent colleague).
7. *Hold off hiring if the practice can be more thriftily covered with episodic or seasonal overtime wages.* Imagine you need an extra tech, but only about 25 hours a week. And you can't find anyone qualified willing to work less than full time. It may be less expensive to pay your current staff overtime when needed.
8. *If the math works, pay a "battle pay bonus" rather than hiring new staff.* Turn to your existing employees and say, "We are now at 40 patients per day and rising. We could either add a new employee to help us on the busiest days, or we could give everyone here a $20 bonus on those clinic days exceeding 48 encounters, if we can do it without a new hire. Which would you prefer?"
9. *Liberalize flexibility.* Staff will often accept a cap on wage hikes if it's traded off for greater flexibility with their hours.
10. *If you only have enough patients to fill up a 4-day week, consider closing the office.* Or at least compress your clinical schedule from 5 days to 4, and bring in a guest subspecialist to help cover overhead.
11. *Shift a larger portion of health insurance costs to employees.* In the typical practice today, staff pay for 30% to 35% of their personal health insurance. If your practice can no longer afford to be more generous that this, shift costs accordingly.
12. *Outsource instead of insourcing.* Or insource instead of outsourcing. It may be more cost-effective to have others outside of your practice handle your dictation or IT support. It may be more cost-effective in a small office to have a staff member stay over after patients leave to handle light office cleaning.

13. *Do not use costly high-level staff for mundane work.* The greenest front-desk staffer, at $14 an hour, can be drafted to run a visual field test; freeing time for a $25-an-hour tech to work up a new patient.
14. *Develop your own staff competence in-house through training programs, rather than hiring expensive, seasoned workers.* This approach is obliged in rural areas with few experienced staff, but urban surgeons can take the same approach. This allows them to save significantly on labor costs and get the added benefit of having staff who learn their way of doing things rather than importing bad habits.
15. *Replace five mediocre workers with three superstars.* The "stars" will cost more per hour, but their aggregate costs will be less, and their output and quality could end up being much higher.
16. *Consider sharing staff with compatible local colleagues.* Even if you practice alone, you may be able to enjoy some of the labor efficiencies of group practice by sharing staff. This could be at relatively junior levels (sharing a receptionist who needs a full-time job, but whom you do not need on Wednesdays) with a practice that could use extra help. Or you could use this approach at very senior levels. As business and regulatory complexities arise, it may be better for two soloists to split the cost of a $90,000 administrator than to pay $60,000 each for a more junior person who is overwhelmed.
17. *Cross-train avidly.* Example: The biggest rookie mistake is to segregate your technical staff into "technicians" who work up patients, "special testers" who test patients, and "scribes" who assist chairside—but who do not cross functional lines with testers or techs. Everyone on the clinic floor should be a "tech-scribe-tester" and float to where they are needed throughout the clinic session.
18. *Think of your staff in terms of "core" and "peripheral."* The core staff (eg, department managers, your administrator) may well deserve above-market wages to reward output and aid loyalty and tenure. To counterbalance these higher costs, you may be able to get by with paying peripheral staff (ie, staff who are more readily replaced) lower-than-market-average wages.
19. *If it becomes necessary, reduce staff wages overall.* If your efforts to shave costs, elevate collections, and sacrifice your personal income are not sufficient, your next recourse will be to cut wages. Just as in patient care, where any strong medicine is likely to have adverse side effects, you will have to plan ahead to mitigate the adverse knock-on effects of a pay cut. Ethically, such efforts should include having the doctors and management staff accept disproportionately higher sacrifices than the rank-and-file.
20. *Make any needed cuts all at once.* When you were 5 years old and your mom had to take off your Band-Aid, she probably—out of kindness—distracted you for a moment and then ripped it off abruptly. It's cruel and disconcerting to staff to have wage freezes and benefits takeaways linger drip-by-drip over several quarters. It's far better to plan out everything that has to be done in a concerted way to bring labor costs into balance, and then get the pain over with all at once.

Do not "frugalize" your practice into the ground. In your zeal to shave staffing costs, do not go too far, reducing care quality or revenue production. And of course, do not let up on efforts to boost provider productivity. If your overall collections—the denominator of the labor cost-percent equation—rise, then labor costs fall in comparative ratio terms.

PS: Since this is a book about being economically effective, realize that you can still use the right-hand two-thirds majority of the bill you clipped for today's exercise as legal tender—just exchange it for an unharmed bill at your bank.

Of Frugality

Health care as an American industry is in the early stages of profound economic transition. Ophthalmic practices are perhaps closer to the cusp than others because of ophthalmology's uniquely measurable outcomes, and because of our high dependency on Medicare entitlement spending.

Allowable Medicare fees, under even the rosiest scenarios, are slated for significant reductions. For the typical general ophthalmologist with a 40% profit margin today, every 1% drop in Medicare fees combined with even mild inflation could result in a 2% pay cut.

Not long ago I launched a collaborative study with several clients on opportunities for "frugal innovation," because profit enhancement—once almost entirely focused on revenue gains—must now simultaneously focus on reductions in the cost to serve each patient.

It now costs the typical general ophthalmology practice well over $100 to transit a single patient visit, including about $50 in lay labor, $10 in rent and utilities, and $5 in marketing costs. As fees erode, one or more of three variables must change to sustain and grow physician income:

1. Practice operating costs must fall.
2. Practice patient volumes must rise.
3. The revenue per average patient visit must grow.

On the cost containment list will be things we never fussed with before. Things like having daytime employees handle light office cleaning throughout the course of the week. Or switching from the sharply creased cotton lab coats the doctors really like, to polyester ones, because the docs can take them home and throw them in the washer instead of paying for dry cleaning. In the future environment, these "picayunish" savings, when added up, will be meaningful.

The term *frugal innovation* arose from one English translation for the Hindi term *Jugaad*, which means an improvised arrangement or work-around obliged by a lack of resources. In India, Jugaad is also the name for a kind of cobbled-together rural vehicle made from a wagon and a repurposed diesel irrigation pump. Crude, ugly, but effective.

Frugal innovation is of course, just another verbal handle—jargon to help drive forward important concepts of doing more faster, more accurately, and consistently, with fewer resources. Many of these code words and associated management frameworks have arisen in industry through the years:

- *Value engineering.* This was launched at General Electric during WWII to overcome shortages of labor and raw materials. In this setting (as in ophthalmology's likely future) necessity was the mother of invention.
- *Kaizen.* After WWII, American consultants in Japan produced a training film *Improvement (Kaizen) in Four Steps.* The term stuck, and was reimported to America.
- *Just-in-time production (JIT).* JIT is generally associated with the Toyota Production System. It was a tactic borne of necessity: Toyota's president said, "Catch up to America within 3 years or Japan's auto industry will not survive." (Sound like ophthalmology?)
- *Lean manufacturing.* This also originated with Japanese manufacturing and was first cited by an MIT student in 1988 in his master's thesis.
- *Six Sigma.* Developed at Motorola in 1986, it became widely known after being applied at General Electric a decade later. It strives to reduce waste by embedding Six Sigma-certified efficiency experts within an organization.
- *Best practice.* This is broadly adopted by business, government, and nongovernmental organizations to accredit the best—or at least a "good"—way of doing things. The American Academy of Ophthalmology's Preferred Practice Patterns are an example.
- *5S.* Perhaps among all of the variously named concepts within the spectrum of frugal innovation, 5S is most immediately applicable to eye care. 5S is yet another workplace organization method developed in Japan, which refers to a list of five actions beginning with the letter "S." As abstracted in Wikipedia, "The list describes how to organize a workspace for efficiency and effectiveness by identifying and storing the items used, maintaining the area and items, and sustaining the new order. The decision-making process usually comes from a staff dialogue about standardization, which builds understanding among employees of how they should do their work."
    - *Sorting.* Eliminate all unnecessary instruments, drops, equipment, and protocols. Go through every inch of your office and remove what is not required. Materials you need most often (eg, forceps and Volk lenses) should be closest at hand.
    - *Straightening out.* Find a place for everything—and that place should be clearly labeled. In an exam room, every drawer and desktop space is segmented and labeled, making it easy to see what's missing or out of place.
    - *Standardizing.* All workstations for a particular job should be identical. All employees doing the same job should be able to work in any station with the same tools that are in the same location in every station. How does this compare to the standards you keep in your pod of exam rooms?
    - *Shining.* Tidy up the workplace periodically and at the end of the day.
    - *Sustaining the practice.* Finally, sustain and continuously improve the new standards you have adopted. Do not allow a gradual decline back to your old standards.

Every business sector is now pursuing frugal innovation, for instance:

- You now pour your own soda at most fast food restaurants.
- Technical support is handled overseas 24/7.
- We now commonly scan and bag our own groceries.
- Toyota now assembles a whole car with just 30 hours of labor. (It still takes some practices up to 3 hours of staff labor to transit a single patient visit.)
- Travel agents once hand-delivered paper airline tickets—not anymore.

Ophthalmology has been at this for a while, too, by:

- Changing from a $20 cataract brochure to a few fact sheets online
- Changing from free patient limo rides to bus tokens for patients
- Changing from $50 postoperative "get well" flowers to a $3 mug—or nothing at all
- Charging up to $115 for a refraction, which was once a bundled fee
- In the future our patients will:
    - Self-appoint online
    - Self-register at a kiosk
    - Get a "ticket" directing them to the appropriate special testing stations
    - Walk themselves from station to station
    - Or they may just step into a local kiosk at the mall to be examined by a doctor in the Philippines or India
    - Or they may refract themselves using a phone app

Beyond Management Slogans: Adopting a Frugally Innovative Mindset

Commercial enterprises—including the smallest ophthalmic practices—become more complex and costly to run as they grow. Bureaucracy and waste creep in by degrees and have to be periodically eliminated. Here's a short list of 50 relatively painless frugal innovations to get you started.

1. Although "frugal" connotes cutbacks, greater profit may sometimes come with looser purse strings: adding a tech allowing you to see more patients, going to a weekend course to learn a new procedure, or elevating one receptionist to "front desk lead" to better coordinate the check-in process.
2. Do the work that change requires. Do not take shortcuts when you see a process or policy that needs to change. Call together all of the involved parties. Agree on the problem and the best revision. Put one person in charge of writing up and implementing the change. Audit for compliance and to ensure that the change is actually working.
3. If you see 60 visits a day, and have only one visual field machine, this probably represents a chokepoint in patient flow. "De-bottleneck" your practice by buying a second field machine (and put it in the same room—it's possible for one tech to run two field exams at a time).

4. Every ophthalmic practice is filled with lots of delicate, expensive equipment that will last longer if given regular service and cleaning. It's easy for all of these service intervals to be forgotten, until a costly repair is required. Keep a master calendar noting all of the major service intervals.
5. Replace your current one-sided printer/copier with a duplex printer to enable printing on both sides of the page.
6. If storage permits, buy in bulk. (But do not spend a dollar on storage used to save a nickel on bulk purchases.)
7. Your practice is your home—and like your real home it's easy for doctors and staff to overlook how shopworn it has become when seen through your patient's eyes. Make a field trip to several eye and noneye offices in your service area. Then return to your office. Is it time for a facelift? It's false economy to not freshen up from time to time.
8. If your accounting firm is still generating your monthly financial statements, shift these in house (it's a snap with QuickBooks) and reserve accounting fees for things you can't do yourself.
9. Over time, or more abruptly if conditions warrant, replace staff whose life circumstances oblige them to work 40 hours each week with more flexible workers who are happy to taper their hours during slow periods, but who can also work 40 hours—even overtime—during your peak season. Beyond the labor flexibility, you will increase the proportion of your staff that work part time and reduce benefits costs.
10. Have a physician take over administrative duties, which empirically can work in a practice with up to about $4 million in revenue, strong mid-level managers, and a committed doctor.
11. Shift 5% of every staff member's compensation to a pay-for-performance arrangement instead of a guaranteed wage.
12. Apply labor substitution. Are you thinking about adding a new member to the team? If you think it's time to add a surgeon, investigate if an optometrist would be more appropriate. This goes all the way down the food chain: Think you need a COT-level tech? Ask, "Would a trainee suffice?"
13. Make all possible vendor payments with cash-back or travel-point credit cards.
14. Find out if you can relinquish part of your existing space to your landlord or sublease it out to a compatible user.
15. Built-in cabinetry work is beautiful, but IKEA may be able to satisfy your needs at a fraction of the cost.
16. The next time you have to replace carpeting, bid out other materials such as ceramic tile. These can be slightly more expensive at the outset, but cost much less in replacement and cleaning over time.
17. Turn all but two private doctor's offices into exam or testing rooms, leaving one private office for the MP and creating a bull-pen office with study carrels for all other providers.

18. The next time you hire a technician, aim for someone who is handy doing minor repairs around the office, which can save the time and cost of outside repairs.
19. If you have a multioffice practice, use the phone and online collaboration tools instead of meeting face to face to reduce travel costs and time for group meetings.
20. Outsource large copy jobs such as forms, staff manuals, and workshop materials for optometric education.
21. E-fax to decrease paper fax use; departments and people receive faxes and directly in their email inbox. (Go to www.efax.com.)
22. Before executing any major loan or lease, confer with your accountant. If you can afford the cash flow differential, it may make sense to buy rather than lease or borrow.
23. Consolidate loans to lock in better terms and potentially ease cash flow constraints. Pay off revolving credit cards monthly, or if credit card debt has ballooned, consolidate and shift to your practice's line of credit to reduce interest costs.
24. Rather than repeating live training sessions, develop videos and written documents for staff skills development. Record a presentation the first time it's given, allowing future staff and those wanting a refresher course immediate access to the material.
25. Hand out occasional taxi and bus passes instead of running a patient transport van.
26. Use a spare room or garage space at home instead of a commercial storage unit.
27. Add motion-sensitive lights in patient lavatories instead of leaving the lights on all day.
28. Have the doctors and administrator share a "unit clerk" or executive assistant instead of using valuable tech time for routine errands.
29. Put every provider and staff member into the same color scrubs, which you order in bulk. It costs more than $15 extra a day (eg, cleaning, wear and tear, shopping time) for a male physician to wear street clothes under a lab coat instead of scrubs.
30. Replace ornate, thirsty office landscaping with xeriscaping. Use silk plants instead of live ones to reduce staff time or plant service costs.
31. Have patients, staff, and providers share unisex bathrooms instead of larger, gender-designated ones.
32. Delay nonessential repairs and maintenance. Patients probably won't notice if you paint the building every 5 years or every 7 years, but over a 30-year practice span, you'll save 28%.
33. Rather than moving into larger office space, hire an ophthalmic space planner to repurpose your existing quarters. Shrink exam rooms. Repurpose your chart room now that we use EHR.
34. Raise the bar for larger, less-than-essential purchases with a purchase requisition system that obliges the person making the order to research alternative options (eg, making do with existing materials, reconditioned rather than new equipment). Enforce a "cooling-off" period for all capital equipment and new hire requests, even requests made by physician-owners.

35. Hold off on developing a satellite office until the full potential of your existing office has been realized.
36. Avoid taking on a low-paying managed care contract unless it's clear that your profit per owner-physician hour will increase by doing so.
37. Frugal innovation is more often a matter of subtraction than addition:
    - On what patients can we omit some exam elements?
    - What is the very least we can put in a cataract surgical tray?
    - Can we simplify and combine office forms?
    - Are there management reports we run that are no longer used to make business decisions?
    - Can we sell, donate, or discard unused equipment and other assets?
    - Are there any memberships we can give up?
38. In the literal sense, get rid of all the junk lying around your office … unused equipment, old brochures you will never use, all the fiddly bits and pieces that accumulate over the years.
39. Do not be the kind of practice administrator or CFO who says, "We spent $120,000 on marketing last year; let's make it $130,000 in next year's budget to keep up with inflation." Start out with $0 on the marketing line, and only add tactics that have a proven value to your practice.
40. Skip all but the smallest *Yellow Pages* ads.
41. Eliminate staffing satellite offices during down times when doctors and patients are not present; roll the phones over to the main office.
42. Do not buy things you do not need and won't use. Remember, anything more than you need is wasted, including:
    - Redundant equipment
    - Software upgrades that do not boost functionality or access to support (and may actually be less stable)
    - Service warrantees for equipment that is unlikely to break down and can be cheaply replaced (like off-the-shelf printers)
    - Professional advice that you are not prepared to implement
    - Annual or monthly fees that can be replaced by an on-call service by the hour or by the project
43. Do not buy things that can be had for free, like tap water (unless your local water is yucky, in which case buy a Brita filter).
44. Review all the ways you use and store paper and look for efficiencies.
    - Do not print out emails unless essential.
    - Even after the shift to so-called "paperless" EHR systems, examine your residual paper trail. It's common to find, even many years after a conversion, practices with electronic records that also make duplicate paper charts, "because the doctors are still not comfortable searching for patient information on a screen." Stop making hard copies of the e-chart for doctors and they will adjust and learn to maneuver through their notes on the monitor.

- Some practices will have clinic patients on EHR, but still use paper records in optical and at the ASC.
- Turn clean, nonconfidential wastepaper into scratch pads.
- Learn how to scan expense reports, vendor invoices, and similar essentials into a readily accessible database.
- Use less-expensive copier paper and disposable towels.
- Use bulk copier paper on a clipboard instead of bound yellow pads.
- Take e-notes on your laptop computer during meetings and read from an agenda on the screen rather than from hard copies.

45. Constantly evaluate optical and contact lens goods costs, which should be under 40% and at or under 50%, respectively. If you have an in-house lab, count all of the costs, including labor, supervision, and floor space, when comparing to the cost-effectiveness of outsourcing.
46. Wherever doctor preferences and standing orders oblige divergent protocols or materials for essentially the same purpose, insist that the providers come up with one agreed, best choice. By eliminating customization, staff training is faster, accuracy increases, and material costs fall when you can lock in bulk orders.
47. Examine associate provider compensation. The market rate today for a better-than-average optometrist working full time in an ophthalmology practice is $150,000 or less, before benefits and taxes. I commonly see doctors with average levels of productivity earning more than $200,000. It is obviously a very delicate task to reset anyone's wages and not be made to feel like an ogre. But, that's what has to be done in the present circumstances.
48. Now and in the future, we are not just running into economic constraints, but also time constraints. Typical managers and MPs have to ration their time carefully for staff meetings, vendor drop-ins, and training. Before you commit your time, ask the following:
    - Will this meeting time be more valuable than the time I am giving up to attend it?
    - Can someone more junior attend this meeting in my stead and synopsize the meeting for me?
    - Is there a more efficient way to accomplish the goals of this meeting, such as a memo, if the main purpose is just to pass along information?
49. Facility development is a rich environment for frugal innovation.
    - You can do with fewer exam rooms and less equipment if you turn each room faster.
    - Exam rooms have been shrinking in size for years—visit the offices of more frugal colleagues to see what you may be able to get away with.
    - A private toilet for each physician is a luxury of the past. (Based on build-out and maintenance costs, and dividing by daily utilization, a surgeon's trip to their personal lavatory costs the company about $5—plus another $12 for every minute off the clinic floor … so hurry-hurry!)

50. Negotiate everything! Most eye surgeons hate confrontation, and they in turn create practice business cultures that avoid negotiating like the plague. It's time to change your mindset in this area, because the ability to negotiate fairly and firmly and with a win-win approach will be a core practice survival skill in the years ahead. It's time to get comfortable with the mild confrontations that will yield you a lower price for the same value, or more value for the same price.

CHAPTER 6

Administration and General Management

Truth is so hard to tell, it sometimes needs fiction to make it plausible.
—Sir Francis Bacon

Of Developmental Hallmarks

An average infant at 6 months of age will reach for an object. At 1 year, the same child will speak a first word. At 2 years, simple phrases and sentences emerge. By age 4, abstract symbols—like d-o-g for dog—are first mastered. And by age 14, with the right teachers and motivation, quadratic equations and Proust. As Mahatma Gandhi wrote, "Constant development is the law of life."

The developmental hallmarks of a child are analogous to the hallmarks of your practice's business operations, except that commercial hallmarks are a function of ***scale,*** not ***age.***

Pinto JB. *Simple: The Inner Game of Ophthalmic Practice Success, Second Edition* (pp 101-128).

Here's an example.

A solo practice typically does not yet have much in the way of a written operations manual—which tends to emerge in a two- or three-doctor practice. A 10-surgeon practice without an elaborate manual is very unusual indeed, and could be thought of as "developmentally lagging."

Childhood development specialists can briskly assess a young patient's developmental hallmarks. Slower development is grounds for intervention. A physical therapist will be brought in to help little Melissa with her lagging fine motor skills, or a speech therapist to help young Matthew with his verbal delays.

What you are probably already looking for in your daily work as a practice leader, consciously or unconsciously, are signs that your practice has outgrown its current operational approaches and needs to move on to intermediate and advanced methods. As the administrator or owner of your practice, part of your job is analogous to the role of a vigilant parent who is constantly on the lookout for developmental lags (and is at the same time proud of any vanguard development).

Here are five developmental practice-business hallmarks for your consideration. Try holding each up as a comparative template for your practice at its current scale, and asking, "For our present size and future aspirations, are we lagging, normative, or vanguard?"

1. A formal, written, long-term ***strategic business plan***
   a. In a small one- to two-doctor practice, there is probably no more than informal discussion about the future, and certainly no formal planning document.
   b. In a three- to five-provider practice, there should reasonably be a brief written document that helps the owners confirm they are all heading in the same direction.
   c. In larger practices, the strategic plan is very much a live, written document that is updated annually and used to prioritize near-term tactics.
2. A formal ***MP*** for the practice
   a. This is obviously moot in a solo practice.
   b. At two or three owners, it's common for the MP role to be more of a figurehead than a formal position.
   c. In larger practices, the MP will commonly spend more than 8 hours a week at the job, have a formal position description, and receive a material financial stipend—it's a real job with really adverse consequences for performance gaps.
3. ***"Office Managers"*** vs ***"Administrators"*** vs ***"CEOs"***
   a. The difference between an OM and an administrator is more than semantics; the former is appropriate to the smallest practices, where the MD-owner is commonly also the chief business officer of the company, and the OM is simply carrying out the policies of the owner, rather than developing their own policies. The OM generally has a "process responsibility" rather than a "profit-and-loss responsibility."

   b. With a bit of growth, a larger practice needs an orthodox administrator—the difference is that this is someone who typically has a freer hand to deploy staff to achieve the board's broad performance goals for the company; they are typically more financially experienced and not as micromanaged as an OM. An administrator has a clearly defined profit and loss responsibility, while still often rolling up sleeves and personally delving into granular operational details.
   c. In the largest ophthalmic practices, we find "CEOs" and "executive directors (EDs)." Such individuals are responsible for the big-picture success of practices ranging to $50 million and more. They have commonly reached a level of their careers where they know the company's financials and performance stats inside and out, but could not post a charge or check in a patient to save their life. (Note: Too-senior an executive in a small practice works just as poorly as having a too-junior manager in a large practice.)
4. ***Middle managers*** and an organized ***management committee***
   a. In small practices, there may be no middle managers at all—everyone reports to the OM or physician-owner; a highly centralized, tooth-of-the-comb organizational structure.
   b. With further growth, the span of control for a central overseer becomes excessive, and mid-level managers or department heads (eg, head tech, billing manager, front desk team leader, optical director) are obliged; developmental lags in this area (ie, not empowering department leads) can hold practices back severely.
   c. With more than 50 lay staff, middle managers must have nearly the same skills and career commitment as the OM does for a smaller practice—they may supervise 10 or more staff members, and they need to meet regularly as a group with the administrator of the practice and the MP to coordinate all the moving parts of a complex enterprise.
5. Performance ***benchmarking***
   a. The smallest, boutique-scaled practices, where everything is simple and in plain sight, can get away with minimal benchmarking, especially if profitability is already high and future goals are modest. A quarterly review of the financial statements and observation of a full reception room every morning confirms that all is well.
   b. Practices making the transition from small to mid-sized commonly get into trouble by not increasing the frequency and depth of their benchmarking. Such practices need monthly financial statements and a monthly flash report showing such key performance indicators as the profit margin, surgical density, average revenue yielded per patient visit, and the average operating cost per visit.
   c. The nation's largest practices—which are typically quite well-run—will track more than 40 normative benchmarks on a regular basis and, because so much is at stake, they will immediately work to reverse any adverse statistics.

In addition to these five gross developmental hallmarks, there are numerous other dimensions, some of which may be more important gauges of progress in your individual setting:

- Accountability documents (eg, project tracking documents, checklists, referral sourcing, comparison with outreach efforts)
- Regulatory awareness and compliance protocols
- Institutional relationships
- The pace of IT and clinical technology adoption
- Marketing and outreach sophistication
- Care pathways, quality assurance, utilization review, and outcomes measurement
- Customer satisfaction tracking

• • •

It's likely as you read through this list that you are already aware of where you are lagging behind. There are several potential drivers for this. Time poverty is the most common—too many projects in the pipeline, compounded by more and more administrative time given over to defensive regulatory oversight instead of offensive business development. Dig deep—your future depends on it.

Of Practice "Birth Defects"

Many years or even decades ago, when your ophthalmic practice was first created, it was likely born with several innate "birth defects"—structural and functional impairments introduced by long-ago staff, accountants, attorneys, and the founders themselves.

Like in a new child, some of these in-born business defects were as easy to see (and as benign) as a child's birthmarks or a funny left earlobe. In your practice, this could be the slightly quirky doctor-founder who is still hanging on, or a penny-pinching philosophy that still holds back growth and retards innovation, while slightly diminishing the quality of patient care—but not enough to cause alarm.

Others founding defects were more serious, and perhaps occult: the business equivalent of a baby's heart anomaly—harmless now, but potentially fatal in the years ahead if not properly treated.

Johann Wolfgang von Goethe wrote in 18th-century Germany, "Certain defects are necessary for the existence of individuality." Without carrying the analogy too far, some of these defects lead to charming differences from one practice to the next, which should be celebrated. Every practice should have its own distinct personality, after all.

However, some of these birth defects, if still present in your practice today, are ripe for revision. Here are six common abnormalities, their origins, their potential for mischief, and their treatment options. Perhaps one or more of these apply to you, your colleagues, and your practice.

1. *An aversion to nominating a doctor-leader.* Bees do it. Wolves do it. Nations do it. So why do so many group practices resist nominating an alpha leader? There are several drivers. In some practices, it's a simple misunderstanding about the role and real value of a MP. In other settings, nobody is willing to step up and commit their time and ego to the task.

But the most common reason is a misplaced desire for absolute equality and to avoid hurting the feelings of those who would not be selected.

Take out your old, legacy partnership or shareholder agreement. It probably called for someone to be a figurehead president, gave them no specific authority, and may have rotated the owners in this position for no more than 1 year at a time. It probably set out no form of compensation for the MP. This is one of the most common—and most disabling—of practice birth defects.

Revision is quite easy: Change your operating agreements if necessary, write a position description for a more enduring MP, and hold an election. MPs should be in place for a minimum term of 2 years, and if they are doing a fine job there need not be any obliged term limits. Depending on the size of your practice, they should receive a stipend of $1,000 to $3,000 per month in most settings—which, given the hours involved, is little more than an honorarium.

2. *Blindness, deafness, and numbness to environmental change.* Most practices operating today were launched in an era where there was relatively little change—and what change there was, was mostly good: The advent of refractive surgery. The development of freestanding surgery centers, allowing a surgeon to double their income per case performed. And the blooming of optical dispensaries, which have boosted typical ophthalmologist incomes about 10%.

   Because change once came mostly slowly and mostly positively, there was really no demand on practice leaders to sniff the wind often for adversity. Until recently, most practice leaders—doctors and administrators alike—were lulled and asleep at the wheel. No longer.

   The happy days of only slow, positive change is over for the current generation. Yes, premium lens technology, the bloom of senior patients, and a few other choice developments will take the edge off. But the prevailing winds will be those carrying fee reductions, intrusions into provider autonomy, and a ballooning of complex regulations.

   Your practice will need a figurative, if not literal, "Chief Change Officer" to help your organization stay upright in the years ahead.

3. *Obliging unanimous consent for every decision in the boardroom.* In the 1960s, 1970s, and 1980s, most new practices were launched as solo shops, often proprietorships, with no corporate structure to speak of. When the typical soloist added their first equal partner, the lawyers created a brief shareholder or partnership agreement. This sparse document often failed to include a tie-breaker mechanism—so every material decision was obliged to be unanimous. This is difficult enough to manage in a two-owner practice—it becomes impossible with a larger group.

   Changing this is easy. Small decisions (eg, a partner buying a new laptop computer) should be at the individual partner's, or even the administrator's discretion, obviously. Mid-size decisions (eg, equipping a new exam lane) should yield to a simple majority. Jumbo decisions (eg, hiring a new provider, terminating the administrator, opening a satellite) should in most settings require the approval of a super-majority, for example four out of five partners.

If you still only have two equal owners, your documents should include a tie-breaker mechanism. This can be a "founder's right" granted to the senior partner—or a right of the higher producer, or the doctor who has the most years left to practice. Quite commonly, residual ties are broken by having the partners agree on an outside tie-breaker, such as the practice accountant for financial questions or the practice attorney for legal ones.

4. *Not spelling out the path to succession.* I suppose it *would* be unexpected for a surgeon whose typical attention span ranges from a 5-minute clinic exam to a 12-minute cataract case to have a short attention span when it comes to long-range planning. That's probably why in about half of the partnership agreements I read nothing is laid out as to an orderly exit strategy.

   This leads to abundant fear, mischief, and discord when the senior partner starts cueing up for their retirement. They expect to get a plump check from the board, and the board counters with, "We'll pay you your pro-rata share of the salvage value of our equipment."

   Pull out your own documents and have a read. They should spell out the following:

   - What happens in the event of a partner's death or disability, their removal at the board's will, or their voluntary withdrawal
   - Specifically, with examples, how the overall practice is valued in each case
   - What portion of the practice each partner owns
   - How a departing partner or their heirs are to be paid, and over what time span
   - If the payments are to be reduced, for example, if a retiring partner gives insufficient notice
   - If there is a ceiling on payout rates (ie, not more than 8% of annual cash flow) so the practice is not crippled when more than one owner leaves at a time

   If not, make an appointment with your attorney this week.

5. *The bad habit of investing every profit dollar into physician compensation.* Some practices are like grandma's muffins: "They squatted to rise, and baked in the squat." In other words, they do not grow as businesses (and muffins) properly should. Why is this? Is the market too competitive? Are the doctors too lazy or unambitious? Usually not. The main reason is underinvestment of profits back into the practice.

   Every practice should have a written business plan. That plan should formally nominate an annual growth pace. And the desired growth pace should, in turn, suggest the level at which you reinvest in the company. It really helps when a board can have the discipline to formally set a minimum floor for such investments. For example, "Because we want to grow our net revenue at 7% per year, a few percentage points higher than the organic growth in local demand for eye care, we realize that we have to withhold 15% of partner income each year from distribution, placing these funds in marketing, practice acquisition, capital projects, and contingency planning accounts."

6. *Not building a management team matched to practice scale and complexity.* Many private practices operating today were set up at a time when peg board systems, carbon paper, and patient ledger cards were state-of-the-art. Profit margins at the outset commonly exceeded 50% and business errors were readily affordable and well-tolerated by a *laissez faire* board. The complexities of LASIK, EHR, RAC audits, MSOs, PPOs, IPAs, and ROIs were not yet invented. The OM was often a family member. The head tech was the oldest staffer or the doctors' pet. And management meetings? Practices could still rely on communications tools of the 1970s, meeting in the hallways and passing messages down the ranks one whisper or growl at a time.

   In the best practices operating today, this legacy of informality has necessarily yielded to formality: an administrator with baccalaureate or better training and an eye for the numbers of the business is needed in most offices today. Lead techs in larger practices need the title (and skill set) of "director of clinical services," and should enjoy hire-and-fire authority over their people. "Billing clerks" have yielded to "revenue cycle managers." All of these lay leaders working in concert with the MP and the board of directors are needed to keep the complex wheels of modern eye care spinning.

Of Administrative Success and Failure

Theodore Roosevelt said that the best executive is the one who has sense enough to pick a good person for the job at hand, and to then have the self-restraint to keep from meddling with them while they do it. He could as well have been talking about good surgeon-owners as executives—and the challenging task of picking the right practice administrator.

Half of all ophthalmic practices in America perform below average, which means that your business has 50/50 odds of being in trouble today. Great practices are built (and flawed practices are fixed) from the top down. After choosing where in the country you want to practice and the right colleagues to practice with, the most important enterprise decision you have as a private practice owner is which lay leader will manage your business.

Lay practice leaders come in five basic flavors:

1. The "chief of staff," who is little more than an executive assistant to an MD owner-operator. Such individuals may receive a salary ranging up to $75,000 or so, and may have the title "manager," but their authority is sharply limited. Everyone really reports to the doctor-boss.
2. The "OM" who (despite the low-octane title) may have full-charge responsibility for a small boutique practice. The OM is typically charged with day-to-day operations but has no material spending or hire-and-fire authority. Depending on the manager's experience and the market, OMs have a base salary today ranging from $60,000 to about $80,000.

3. The “administrator” is a kind of “CEO-lite” responsible for both operations and profitability, but in most cases with relatively limited off-budget spending authority. The vast majority of ophthalmic practices in America today, being in the $2 million to $5 million bandwidth, employ a person they call an administrator. What does that cost them? In rural America, the administrator of a large practice may earn less than the OM of an urban practice—but the wide-ranging base salary for experienced administrators today is $60,000 to $150,000.
4. The “ED,” who typically leads practices with revenue in the range of $5 million to $20 million, is predictably hard-charging and career-focused. In alignment with the MP, they take command of the practice boardroom … and are often granted a much higher level of discretionary spending than more junior administrative colleagues. EDs pull in $100,000 to $200,000 as a base wage—not because the title is more impressive than an administrator's, but because the ED's skill sets and personal commitments are higher. A $10 million practice needs four times the leader of a $5 million practice.
5. The “CEO” is generally found in only the largest practices. They are granted significant executive and financial authority over the practice. CEOs cue up long-term strategies and budgets for final board approval and, if they are the right person in the right job, their board need only provide light-handed oversight, not fiat control. The highest-paid ophthalmic executives today enjoy physician-level base salaries ranging to $300,000 and perquisites taking this figure much higher.

As you can see from this, no matter if you have a small or large practice, you are going to have to spend about 1% to 5% of cash flow to hire and support the brains of the outfit.

With that kind of money at stake, you want to find the right kind of leader-manager, someone suited to the scale and aspirations of your practice. It is as big an error to undershoot and select a junior executive assistant to run a large practice as it is to overshoot and hire a CEO for a small-time operation.

Here are some considerations to help you get it right the first time around:

- The hardest practice to manage is the mid-sized practice. You have to know how to do every job in the practice and have a balanced portfolio of leadership and management skills. Small, solo practices have fewer moving parts and are relatively easy to manage. Enormous practices, captained by CEOs and EDs, have a deep bench of middle managers with lots of redundant in-house skills and are comparatively easy to manage (even if they are often difficult to lead.)
- Decide whether you need more of a leader, more of a manager, or a blend of the 2. Leadership and management are overlapping and complimentary, but very different skills. This is frustratingly evident in the functioning of most elected officials. The leadership chops needed to stand up and charismatically frame up a mission and pull people along in that direction has little correlation to getting the job done. In personnel management circles, a great leader who speaks well, but can't perform, is called a “communicative incompetent.” Do not hire one of these.

- No administrator has a complete skill set. Some are excellent at personnel issues, but weak at finance. Some are weak at marketing, but a wiz at operating efficiencies. Know your prospective administrator's core competencies before you make the hire and realize that any missing skills will either have to be learned, supplied by someone else in the practice, or outsourced.
- The core competencies of the administrator you hire should coincide with your practice's greatest current and anticipated needs. If you're financially on the ropes, you need numeracy. If referral source outreach is flagging, you need selling skills. If customer service is your weakest link, make sure your new hire has a proven record of improving service performance in a similar setting.
- Practice management and leadership is only partially a so-called "learned" profession. Unlike law, engineering, or medicine, there is no agreed or obliged standard of licensure, no test to pass. Even if you personally have a great educational pedigree, do not be an academic snob. I've seen more MBAs blow up practices than up-through-the-ranks managers with associate degrees.
- Hiring a high-energy, gung-ho person to lead your practice is necessary, but insufficient. To increase the odds of business success, one needs to hire gung-ho people who have a proven track record of analogous performance in analogous settings. Hiring an ex-hospital administrator for your very large practice may sound logical, but the skill set needed to run a 400-bed hospital is profoundly different than the skills needed to run even the largest ophthalmology practice.
- Executives who are gung-ho but inexperienced, when paired with a high-demand boss who labels all requests "RED HOT," will collect more open, incomplete projects than closed accomplishments. If you are a high-demand practice owner, make sure you hire someone who can prioritize and stand up to your criticism about why last week's hot project hasn't been launched yet.
- Big brains are obligatory in your top executive. But intelligence is an incomplete substitute for raw time commitment. Great administration is more often a matter of working harder than working smarter.
- Beyond the time commitment of your administrator, the MP of the practice must commit time and attention to the company. Even the strongest CEOs of the largest practices in America (that I see firsthand) struggle if their lead MD counterpart is time-poor or disengaged. In practical terms, this typically translates to the effective MP of a solo to five-owner practice spending up to 8 hours a week on leadership duties, and the MPs of larger practices commonly putting in 12+ hours a week.
- Management and leadership are contact sports. To be successful and achieve the shortest cycle time between finding and fixing a problem, everyone who touches each problem has to be in the same room together. Ideally, in a group practice with numerous providers, the doctors' personal offices (or study carrels in thrifty practices) are arrayed around a large board table, and the administrator's private office is in this same suite. An executive assistant, bookkeeper or CFO, and IT exec are nearby. This increases the odds of owners and managers running into each other throughout the day, therefore developing stronger relationships and applying better solutions to problems they find faster.

• • •

No Administrator Lasts Forever

Not all human pairings work out over the long haul. Half of all marriages unwind. Only about half of the eye surgeons brought in as owner-track associates actually stick around and become a partner. Your average practice lay staffer will leave you after just 4 years on the job. And virtually all of your acquaintances will fade away well before you grow old, even in the age of Facebook.

Nowhere in the sphere of your practice is this excess human churning more costly and frustrating than with your practice's administrator, whose average tenure in the average setting is about 6 years, more or less.

Based on my experience, about 40% of practice owners reading this are ecstatic about their administrator or practice manager. Another 50% or so are equivocal or worse. Approximately 10% are in the hunt for a new lay leader, or will be within the next year.

These feelings can wax and wane. For many surgeons reading this, a love-hate relationship has existed for years between you and your lay staff leader. You're often saying to yourself: "They are too good to fire, but too (insert adjective of your choice here) to keep on the payroll."

Let's explore 10 signals that it may be time to terminate or demote your current OM, administrator, ED, or CEO.

1. *Trust has been breached.* This first signal is impossible to quantify. It's a feeling thing. Such feelings can be sparked by one obvious ethical lapse (like letting a personal expense slip onto the company credit card) or an accretion of small items adding up over time. When the "distrust score" is over a given mark—and all of us have different tolerance and forgiveness levels in this area—the manager has to go.
2. *Your practice has outgrown your manager.* Managers and their practices should be a closely matched pair. Ideally, as the practice grows in complexity, your administrator will grow in competency. Sometimes the practice is static while the administrator blooms, in which case the administrator should be the one to leave to find new horizons. Just as often, the practice grows at a faster pace than the manager. If your otherwise valued administrator is unable to keep up, it may be time for a change. This may require nothing more than some educational time at the national meetings, coursework, a more engaged physician-leader, or the engagement of outside expertise.
3. *Your practice is stale because your manager is stale.* In an ideal world, the administrator and lead physician are a dynamic duo, keeping the company fresh and acting as a pacer for each other when one or the other gets stale. Your practice is a living organization. To be successful it needs to feed on the ideas and energy of its leaders. If your administrator is burned out or has simply been drained of creative juices by too many years in the same position, it may be time for a change.
4. *Your manager's numeracy is not up to contemporary requirements.* In days gone by, the acceptable core competencies to run an eye clinic were things like product knowledge, an instinct for managing people, or marketing. Today, the number one competency required is numeric skills (followed closely by clear written and oral communication and raw endurance). If your current manager is, "Um, like, not

really into math," it may be time to make an exchange for someone more numerate, or to at least buttress any weakness in this area with an in-house accounting or bookkeeping resource.

5. *Practices are merging, and only the strongest manager is needed going forward.* This one is pretty straight forward, and as soon as merger talks commence in earnest, both managers should pretty much know the score. In some cases, the leadership role can be shared, at least through an initial period of operations consolidation. But in most settings a zero-sum choice is obliged, with one winner and one loser. Have the ethical compass to make your choice early and help the loser find a new position in the community.
6. *Interpersonal conflicts have risen to the breaking point.* If you live with a teenager (or act like one in your off hours), you probably know all about "life points"—scores you build or shrink based on your success in a video game. Administrators play the same game, only in real life. They start a new job in your practice with 100 points. Then they lose points whenever they argue with you unpleasantly or make a mistake, and gain points with critical accomplishments. Lose too many points and a manager is pink-slipped—or in many cases should be.
7. *Your present manager is good—but you've discovered someone who is great.* Unlike romantic relationships, a roving eye is good for business, and it's perfectly acceptable to trade up every once in a while. Even when you're not looking, you may run across a manager so superior and such a great fit with the needs of your practice that it trumps your loyalty to your present administrator. When this happens, do the right thing. Give your otherwise great outgoing manager significant notice, a generous severance package, and abundant support in their job search.
8. *Your manager's life situation no longer allows a focus on your practice.* Life changes. Your manager may have domestic wobbles, start a family, or start taking care of an ailing parent or spouse. If there is a new personal challenge to manage, this can take away a critical slice of management time and attention needed to commit every week to your company. Such a distraction may be permanent or just temporary. (Offering a last chance to get back in the game or a leave of absence may be more appropriate in these situations than frank termination.)
9. *Your practice is faltering, you do not know why, and your administrator isn't struggling by your side to turn things around.* Ideally, you're in this together. If your practice is on the skids and you feel like you're more engaged with the turnaround than your manager is, talk about it. If on most days you still feel like the only sled dog pulling in the harness, it may be a signal to find another manager.
10. *Practice revenue is shrinking, and economics no longer warrant a higher-level executive.* This is rare today, but we may see more of this in the future. If you have a high-priced administrator and your top-line collections are shrinking, it may be necessary to downsize the cost of your "brains" to fit new circumstances. In the future we may see a trend in smaller practices. This has been long observed in optometry, where an engaged physician-owner takes over running day-to-day operations. Experience shows this is not ideal, but it can work fine for selected providers in selected settings, and acceptably well in practices up to about $4 million in annual collections.

These are 10 reasonable reasons to consider terminating your administrator. There is at least an equally long list of reasons to ***not*** terminate, and I've seen all of these in the eye care boardrooms of America, including:

- *One-time errors and omissions.* Remember that although you may hold yourself to standards of near perfection as a provider, the rest of the world is human. One or two crummy management decisions a month is par for the course.
- *Firing as a result of scrupulous honesty about bad news.* You want to create an environment where your administrator doesn't fear for their job because of speaking the truth.
- *Failure to recognize that no manager has a 100% complete skill set.* Strong financial managers may need outside help for marketing, IT, or human resource expertise.
- *Letting things build up in silence—failure to confront your manager in the moment when they disappoint you.* You should give your administrator ongoing feedback—plus and minus—about performance so that over time you'll get more of what you like and less of what you dislike.
- *Failure to provide progressive discipline.* Rather than lowering the boom abruptly in response to poor performance on the part of any staffer, corrective action should be taken in stages (eg, verbal warnings, written warnings, formal retraining, wage reductions).
- *Judging your manager's job performance based on affability or lack thereof.* There are plenty of communicative incompetents in every industry who should be weeded out. There are also a lot of relatively dry, dour—but administratively brilliant—business leaders out there in the world of ophthalmology. As a practice owner, it pays to know the difference and not sack an otherwise committed executive just for not smiling or asking you to lunch every day.

Of Patient Satisfaction

He profits most who serves best.
—Arthur F. Sheldon

What do you and your practice sell, really? Aside from objective clinical and surgical outcomes—such as greater comfort, blindness averted, and optimal sight—***patient satisfaction*** is the core "product" of your practice.

A high level of patient satisfaction pays numerous dividends:

- Complaints are lower, reducing staff stress and freeing up their time for other duties.
- Established patients stay with the practice, reducing the high cost of recruiting new patients.
- It costs about $500 to recruit a new patient with direct-to-consumer advertising—satisfied patients tell their friends about your practice *for free.*
- Happy patients create a positive feedback loop, spurring the referral behavior of their optometrists and physicians.

- Satisfied patients invest more trust in your care, giving their consent for needed services more readily, reducing patient education time, and making it easier to broaden your scope of care.
- Satisfied clinical patients stay in the practice and purchase optical goods and elective services; they do not have any reason to shop around for alternatives.
- When your patients are truly satisfied with your care as a physician, including the mechanics of their transit through your office, your professional life is more personally rewarding, which can extend your career life and make retirement easier.

Always do more than is required of you.
—General George S. Patton

What elevates patient satisfaction? The list is enormous and limited only by your resources, empathy, and imagination. One client has a glass-fronted refrigerator with free drinks. In another office they have a rule: "Never say 'No' to a patient, no matter what they ask." A third ophthalmologist calls every new patient the next day to see if there were any overlooked questions from the most recent visit.

Excess waiting time is the number one complaint of patients about their doctor visits. In ophthalmology, the primary waiting time (the time from on-time arrival to rooming of the patient) should not exceed 20 minutes. The total transit time for a routine visit should not exceed 70 minutes. If your patient flow timelines materially exceed these upper limits, conduct a time study and engage your entire practice team to compress the visit to patient-expected bounds.

How do we know that we're getting things right and that everything we're doing is enough? We have to continuously measure patient satisfaction.

The world's largest businesses take customer care seriously, hiring academic research specialists to dissect the nuances of their service-value proposition. Every customer service action and public word uttered by the Fortune 500 is parsed for its contribution to a happy customer. Staff are scripted to say and do the right thing at the right time, at every point in the transaction.

Of course, no private medical practice has the resources to evaluate customer satisfaction to this depth or level of statistical formality. You must take a guerilla approach to customer research, just as you have learned be a guerilla fighter when it comes to your overall marketing tactics. Most practices stop short at brief written surveys, and call the job done. They hand out survey cards at checkout or email follow-up questionnaires to a cross-section of patients.

Written surveys like this are of limited value in understanding customer satisfaction. They can certainly help to objectify just what many patients feel about one issue or another—for example, to identify what portion of your patients feel that waiting time is appropriate vs excessive. But written surveys are notoriously less useful at identifying actionable problem areas in the first place. As the typical small practice owner or manager, this is the most important information to gather.

Written surveys suffer a variety of shortcomings, the largest of which is an adverse selection of respondents—only your raving fans and your biggest disparagers tend to respond. In addition, written surveys do not allow patients to elaborate much on their feelings and can't draw out very creative suggestions for your operational problems.

For a deeper understanding of your practice's ability to satisfy patients, phone surveys are vastly superior. A so-called "laddering" survey (ie, think: "I'm climbing down a ladder into this patient-customer's mind") will allow you to explore in depth how you're doing.

Here's a simple protocol.

Before starting, make sure that you have provider buy-in and approval of the process. The results of this survey protocol will almost always include negative comments from some patients about their doctor. If you spring any negative survey results on an unsuspecting doctor, without providing the advance courtesy of reviewing the protocol, it's understandable why that doctor will reject the findings.

Depending on how serious you are about the study, select between 5 and 20 patients at random per provider per month, whom your practice has seen in the past month. Select a surveyor to place the calls—this can be the practice administrator, the marketing director, or an outside party—it shouldn't be someone who is likely to be overly attached to the outcome of the study, or have their feelings hurt (eg, do not use a physician's spouse, a receptionist, or a technician). Call each selected patient and pursue the following introduction:

> Hello, this is Mary from Dr. Susan Smith's office, your eye doctor. Each month we randomly select a few patients we've recently served to find out what kind of a job we're doing here at Smith Eye. I'll only need a few minutes of your time, if you can help us out.

With the patients' approval, you can then pursue a line of questioning that covers their global experience with the clinic:

- How easy was it making an appointment?
- Did we provide you with a reminder call?
- Was it easy finding the office and getting a place to park?
- Describe your experience checking in with the front desk.
- Were you seen on time, or did you feel like your initial wait was excessive?
- Tell me what kind of a job the technician, the staff member who first worked you up, did.
- How did your time with the doctor go? Did they answer all your questions? Address your chief concerns?
- At checkout time, were you clear about when you should next come back for an appointment? Did the fees seem fair and reasonable?
- Is there anything else we could have done more of, less of, or differently to make your total experience better?

With a cooperative interview subject and an adroit interviewer, these sessions can last 10 to 15 minutes or longer. Write down each patient's responses and collate the results monthly.

Implement any obvious improvements. Discuss material failings, privately in many cases, with the relevant parties (ie, take a technician aside and tell them how patients are mentioning how they are too abrupt sometimes).

Repeat the survey at appropriate intervals for each provider. The frequency and depth of such interviews should be proportional to the quality of patient care and caring you are providing. If your practice has lots of problems, increase the survey frequency—if you have few problems, you might only need to repeat this survey protocol a couple of times a year.

• • •

Do you think this is going overboard? That your staff would never have time to call a few patients a month? Consider this. I've owned a Toyota 4-Runner for many years. Toyota is famous for the satisfaction level of its customers. When I take this SUV into the local dealership for routine service it sets me back about $75. Invariably I'm called within 24 hours by a customer service rep who asks, "How did we do?"

If a $200 billion company can call every customer it serves about their $75 oil change, can't you do the same for a very small cross-section of your clinical and surgical patients?

Of Coaching Points From Managers to Physicians

In the midst of a daylong managers' workshop, we once asked participants to write down and turn in a short answer to a difficult, highly charged question: "What are some things that the doctors in your practice do that hold back the growth and development of your organization?"

The audience responses following will come as no surprise to those who are practice management veterans, but may shock some physician readers:

- *A lack of teamwork.* This was the most common catch-all criticism, which ranged from not responding to emails or following agreed-upon rules to the point of being baldly dishonest. Examples shared included doctors saying "Yes" in the boardroom or to the administrator, and then undermining on the clinic floor what was agreed. Some doctors were described to be changing policies without telling others. A central theme expressed was concern about an all-too-common double standard: doctors (especially owners) not personally demonstrating the kind of work habits and team-building behaviors that are expected of lay staff. These behaviors include arriving late to clinic, hoarding charts, and giving certain staff the cold shoulder while lavishing undue praise on favorites. One respondent wrote: "Our doctor discounts obviously valuable staff members, while inflating the value of others who do not deserve his praise."
- *Poorly developed communication skills.* Providers were cited for jumping to conclusions without listening to all sides, finishing other people's sentences for them, butting heads with management rather than communicating more productively … and especially a hesitancy to confront or engage in difficult conversations.
- *Being rude, condescending, and belittling with staff.* Some providers were described as seeming to derive pleasure in finding fault with others and meting out criticism that is out of proportion with the scope of a given problem. One participant wrote,

"We are so afraid of what he's going to say next that we go out of our way to not talk to this doctor at all." Another wrote, "Our doctor is very kind and appropriate with patients, yet is rude and inconsiderate with staff members. Sometimes such behavior can be consistent, but it's more often unpredictable and presents as frequent mood swings. Blaming and fault finding. Arrogance."

- *Unreasonable expectations.* An example cited was a variety of perfectionistic behaviors; a disconnect between demanding high performance from the team, while not being willing to release the resources required to staff up to needed levels.
- *Overt "anger management" issues.* This is always a serious problem, but is particularly adverse when it takes place in front of patients.
- *Being inconsistent and indecisive from day to day.* For example, "My doctor has an inability to plan ahead and think about the future." Eye care is typically provided in 5-minute units from room to room, so it's not unusual for doctors to be lost in the now rather than thinking a year down the track and anticipating future needs.
- *Old-fashioned selfishness.* This manifests as not considering the needs of others; a "me first" approach to all practice decisions.
- *Excess controlling behavior.* For example, "One of our doctors is a control freak." Being a know-it-all. Negative reactions to new ideas unless they came from the offending provider.
- *Passive-aggressive behaviors.* Pot-stirring—"If a crisis isn't brewing, our doctor will create one."
- *Being suspicious, to the point of paranoia.* Trust is a vital component of working groups if they are to function effectively, and trust has to be built from the top of the organization.
- *Disengagement with and disinterest in staff and their lives.* This issue is one of degrees. Too much or too little engagement with support staff can be problematic. A "Goldilocks" approach is indicated, which requires judgment, sensitivity, and setting limits.
- *Defensiveness (and an inability to accept constructive coaching).* Insecure people (and many physicians are less secure than they should be, given their intellect and training) tend to be resistant to feedback.
- *Lazy work habits on the part of young doctors.* Some time ago I coined the term "precocious sweatophobia" to describe the habits of some young providers who are curiously less workaholic than the previous generation. When a young provider with commendable work–life balance replaces a retiring high-volume senior doctor, this can create headaches for administration and frank financial collapse for the practice.
- *An "ADHD-like" distractibility.* Respondents described this in a lot of ways: "An inability to stay on task ... a poor sense of time ... procrastination ... poor time management ... thinking in distracted, round-about terms ... and out loud rather than forming his thoughts privately and then directing staff or patients clearly ... asks for management to research something and then ignores the findings as though he's forgotten he ever asked for the help ... tells multiple staffers to do the same task ... gives conflicting orders to two different staff members."

- *Overt discourtesy to patients.* Examples of this are answering personal cell phone calls in the exam room, arriving late for clinic, and blowing off reasonable patient questions.
- *Being overcommitted.* Taking on too many projects at once and performing them poorly or not at all.
- *Paperwork gaps.* Attendees wrote: "Coding 'any old way' instead of what's correct ... holding onto charts ... not finishing chart entries at the time of an individual exam, but instead pushing all of the notes and dictation to the end of the day ... multiweek delays with dictation."
- *An unrecognized need to retire.* One person wrote: "Our surgeon's skill is getting shaky and he's getting forgetful ... hard to tell him this, though."

The late, great comedian George Carlin said, "Men are from Earth. Women are from Earth. Deal with it." Maybe it's just the ophthalmologists who are from an alien planet. They certainly act that way from time to time. If you are a physician and recognize yourself in any of these comments, sit down with your administrator and start a dialogue on how you might improve.

Of Provider Performance Reviews

It's odd, isn't it? The doctors working up and down the hall in your clinic have each spent a quarter of a century in school, receiving along the way thousands of test grades and report cards reflecting their performance in hundreds of classes. And yet, if you are like the average employer or leader of ophthalmologists, you're shy about sitting down once or twice a year with a recap of each doc's strengths and weaknesses.

When I ask providers—associates and partners alike—to whom they formally report in their practice, they'll commonly give me a blank stare. Then they say something like, "Now that I think of it, I'm not sure. Nobody, I guess."

All of a practice's providers should live formally an organization chart and report to *somebody.* They might report to the MP (or another designated owner) for clinical issues or, in a very large practice, to the medical director.

Every associate provider, whether on a partner track or a durable employee, should ideally be reviewed twice a year. But even partners should receive formal feedback at least annually.

Annual Formal Feedback

What should you measure? The short answer to this question in your unique practice is probably a pretty long one: everything you can think of that reflects a dimension of what is important to you and your practice. The list should be broken down into categories. Here's a starter list of 21 elements for you to consider. Eliminate items that are not important to you. Add performance dimensions that are important in your unique setting. This could include research or teaching, wider community involvement or committee leadership within the practice, or a measure of the associate's overall fit with the culture of your practice.

Comprehensive Professional Standards

1. *Timeliness.* What it takes most to be a great worker, as the saying goes, is just showing up on time. Also, does the provider complete charting, dictation, and project commitments on time with a minimum of staff reminders?
2. *Patient care and caring.* You can lump this together, or break it up into several subcategories:
   a. Clinical and surgical judgment and decision making
   b. Adherence to agreed care pathways
   c. Treatment and surgical outcomes
   d. Complications management and outbound referrals
   e. Communication with patients and family members
   f. General affability and the ability to bond with patients
3. *Conflict resolution.* Being open to difficult conversation. Being fearless about telling the truth early rather than withholding difficult news (eg, about a patient the associate may have made unhappy).
4. *Absence of drama.* Quells rather than passing along and amplifying rumors—doesn't magnify small problems, imagined slights, or the daily irritations of clinical practice. Doesn't storm down the hall when things do not go their way.
5. *Avoids support staff fraternization.* Maintains a professional but friendly distance with lay support staff.
6. *Practice knowledge.* Maintains an intimate understanding, enhanced over time, of the various services provided by the practice, their prices, success drivers, and profit dynamics.
7. *Attention to detail.* An extreme attention to operational detail and smooth daily operations is required in a complex and changing environment where inattention may cost someone's sight.

Leadership

8. *Models appropriate professional behavior and helps build a foundation of leadership.* Consistently demonstrates the ability to build and lead a senior staff team, and to actively mentor and coach not only departmental leaders but junior providers.
9. *Planning and development.* Participates in the preparation (and at least annual review) of the practice's strategic and business operations plan; leads or delegates the revision process for each subsequent edition.
10. *Committee/board positions.* When invited, is an effective member or observer in the boardroom and effectively supports the practice's various standing committees.
11. *Career commitment.* Meets and exceeds the basic time requirements of the position, including occasional demands for evening and weekend meetings.
12. *Recruitment.* Involved from time to time in provider and senior staff recruitment activities.

Productivity

13. *Overall productivity.* When there is a lull in patient volumes, uses time effectively (eg, answering priority phone calls, completing dictation, returning email).
14. *Volumetric performance.* Meets or exceeds reasonable expectations for the number and type of patients seen … gracefully accepts work-ins and emergency appointments.
15. *Financial performance.* Is on track with agreed hallmarks for collections and profit contribution.
16. *Resource utilization.* Uses staff, equipment, and facility resources to their best purposes; is reasonable about asking for new resources, but has an understanding that not every equipment request will be honored.
17. *Referral behavior.* Refers preferentially, when appropriate, to in-house subspecialists rather than outside providers—supports ancillary services (eg, ASC, special testing, optical, low vision, audiology)
18. *"Coachability."* Is approachable and eager to obtain constructive input from colleagues and support staff, is nondefensive, and readily adopts reasonable corrective actions.
19. *Sensitivity to cost containment.* Actively looks for opportunities to reduce the cost of providing patient services, without eroding care quality.
20. *Contributes to operational enhancements.* Makes suggestions to improve practice workflow. Aids with periodic revisions to the practice operations manual.
21. *Risk management.* Supports the practice's efforts to reduce malpractice and other liability. Uses good judgment to suspend or revise any clinical or business practices believed to be inappropriate.

Develop a Scoring System

Every grading system needs a scale. Once you have decided what elements to measure, you can use the familiar ABCDF scale, or count up from 1 (low) to 5 (high). Here's an example:

5 Outstanding performance—Consistently exceeds standards
4 Above standards—Frequently exceeds standards
3 Meets standards
2 Below standards—Infrequently meets standards, improvement is needed
1 Unacceptable performance—Significant improvement is urgently required

Do not just score your providers in one direction. Ask them to score themselves as well, using the same tool that you develop using these ideas as the jumping-off point. If you need another opinion or two before you sit down for the review, ask for input from your practice's head tech, ASC director, optical manager, or other well-placed and thoughtful individuals.

Of Marketing and Selling

Marketing, to get us all off on the right foot, is one of the most confusing, underappreciated, complex, vexing, bungled, and unaccountable dimensions of business management. But marketing, for all its frustrations, is vital to practice survival— much less success, now more than ever. Every practice "markets" (well or poorly, whether they know it or not) and all practices, even ones that are good at marketing, waste at least half of their promotional budget every year. They rarely know which half.

Although markets have been changing drastically in eye care for the last generation, the definition of marketing stays the same. Marketing is nothing more, and nothing less ***than establishing and maintaining exchange relationships with customers.***

These "customers" come in a wider array than just patients, of course. Customers also include affiliates of patients (ie, the daughter who brings her mother in for cataract surgery … and perhaps helps her pay for lens upgrades), distributors of your care (including all manner of referral sources), and third-party payers.

Ever since 1977, when the US Supreme Court reversed efforts by the Arizona State Bar to prohibit professional advertising, doctors in America have had the same opportunity as any other vendor to build their businesses through open promotion. And among doctors, ophthalmologists have been in the vanguard of both marketing expenditures and marketing sophistication. This has occurred for a number of reasons:

- Ophthalmology has a wider array of services than most other specialties—there is more to promote and get the word out about.
- Ancillary opticals and surgery centers, providing passive income, represent a strong incentive to build market share and patient volumes.
- Patients can still self-refer for most eye care services, so a direct-to-consumer approach can be used. Many of these services are elective and paid for out of pocket.
- Ophthalmology is a relatively competitive field, with an excess of providers in many markets.
- Ophthalmology is a largely fixed-cost business. If you're in a 500 patient-per-month practice, the profit margin derived from seeing patient number 501 is nearly 100%—so it's easy to justify material outlays for practice-building.
- Relationships with patients in eye care are generally longitudinal. Gaining a new patient is on average not just another exam or procedure this year, but an annuity stream that can represent tens of thousands of dollars. This substantiates marketing outlays that are a lot higher than in practices that treat brief disease episodes and then discharge their patients.
- The significant co-management intersect of ophthalmology and optometry is not present in any other specialty; this form of marketing is uncommon in other specialties.
- Ophthalmology is a financially robust domain of medicine; there are more discretionary dollars available for experimenting.
- Ophthalmology is an unusually well-connected specialty of medicine, with strong communication ties criss-crossing the nation. What works, marketing-wise, in one market is rapidly shared around the national, even international community.

Let's discuss what's working in ophthalmic marketing today in broad terms. And then let's also talk about what flops.

Internal Marketing

We always need to start with *internal* marketing before considering *external* promotion. How's your current practice "product?" So-so? Awesome? Really pretty bad? Remember that nothing makes a flawed practice fail faster than great external promotion.

Your facility is the "packaging" for what you're trying to sell. You can be the most credentialed and caring provider in the world, but patients won't come—or at least come back—if your office quarters are shabby. As a general guide, let's do what hotel chains have done in recent years. Even down-market and mid-market chains, if they're successful, have great curbside appeal, adequate parking, and a nice lobby. It's perfectly okay to have the guest rooms be a little "industrial" so long as the front end of the outfit has sufficient swank.

Signage should be as large and well-lit as local ordinances will allow. Signs should include provider names and principal services. If you are able to mount a sign large enough to accommodate a changeable marquee, all the better. Change the copy every week—driving by and seeing "Floaters and Spots Mean Your Retina's Kaplotz" will get a lot more attention (and patients) than a tasteful, unlit brass plaque on the door.

Doctor appearance and affability are key. ***You*** are your practice's product. And you are judged at every turn. Do you have a nice photograph on your website? Are you well-groomed? Do you dress successfully? Do you greet patients warmly? Remember some point of trivia from their last visit? Address the chief complaint? Provide ample reassurance and praise? Treat staff like respected colleagues within earshot of patients? Often provide a reassuring, bonding touch?

Stunning customer service by lay staff is paramount and can make up for almost any facility gaps—even doctors' deficits. Your staff members are responsible for far more patient contact than you. Formal, ongoing efforts to hire friendly staff and continuously inspire great customer service are critical, even in the smallest practices.

Recall and continuity of care work constitutes great medicine, great medico-legal prophylaxis, and incredibly effective marketing. If your established patient base is not growing roughly in synch with the number of new patients, your practice is leaking customers. External marketing in such settings is like bailing a leaking boat instead of simply patching the hole.

The secret weapon of internal marketing is for you, as the doctor, to overtly ask every patient to refer to you. Every departing patient should be handed three cards with the phrase, "Please tell your friends about the importance of regular eye care."

External Marketing

Your practice will be more successful with a "brandable" name. "Curtiss Eye Care" is a unique, branded name. "Hudson Valley Eye Care" is generic and not very brandable. "Curtiss" will have to spend less than "Hudson" promotionally to get the same name recognition.

Although paid advertising in general/geriatric care settings has diminished somewhat with the drop-in allowable fees, there is still an important role for such promotion. In the right market, with the right message, and the right long-term commitment, advertising—especially testimonial ads—are still effective.

Publicity has emerged as an important adjunct to ever-more-expensive paid advertising for larger practices, which have interesting stories to tell. The larger the market, the more you have to turn to a seasoned local publicist for support.

Your website and associated social media efforts will continue to outshine old-school media advertising as a return on investment. Mass print and electronic media are not dead, but in the years ahead, we will be vastly more dependent on the internet for all age groups than legacy communication channels.

The savviest practices have tapered their *Yellow Pages* advertising down to whatever comes free with their commercial phone numbers.

Building and sustaining your refractive surgery practice continues to require much more sophistication and budgetary support than any other eye care practice segment. It is common for old-line practices to spend very little on direct-to-consumer marketing, while relative newcomers to LASIK commonly spend 10% to 20% of their meager refractive surgery revenue. In today's tough, down market, you have to get price, product, and promotion precisely right—for many years; and even then local nuances, provider tenacity, and luck are the critical co-factors. With aging boomers shifting to lens-based vision correction, LASIK isn't going to fade away, but it also won't be a growth segment.

The advent of premium cataract lens options (PIOLs) has opened a whole new world of promotional demands and opportunities. The most aggressive practices have been doing well in this new sphere, implanting PIOLs at twice or more times the average national rates. Those practices that a generation ago were successfully building elective refractive, plastics, and primary care businesses are the same practices that today lead in the percent of cataract patients opting for surgical upgrades.

Marketing Budgets

Subspecialty, referral-based practices need spend very little on overt marketing, aside from outreach and a few special events throughout the year. As a very general rule of thumb, an established/general/geriatric practice with modest growth goals in a benign market with little competition can get by spending 1% to 3% of annual collections on marketing. If your market is tougher, or your growth goals are higher, you may need to spend 3% to 5%.

The Biggest Marketing Errors

There are many more ways to get marketing wrong than to get it right. Here is a checklist of the most common errors:

- *A lack of goals.* You should know what specific, numeric outcomes you desire from your marketing efforts in financial, case volume, and market share terms.
- *A mismatch between goals and resources.* You probably can't build practice revenue by 15% a year when you are spending 1% of revenue on marketing.
- *Inadequate staying power.* It can take years to build traffic. Typically, just about the time you get sick and tired of seeing your own ads is when they are just starting to register with the public.
- *Spreading your budget too thinly.* You can't take on numerous marketing projects with a limited budget. It is better to do one or two core tactics well.
- *Inexperienced advice.* While it's unlikely you'll find a seasoned eye care marketing expert in your hometown, try to at least work with someone who is experienced in health care or service-sector marketing. It's easy to waste a fortune on fees teaching your local, well-meaning marketing firm all about how health care works.
- *No customer research.* You must survey and poll customers and prospective customers avidly to find your next opportunities.
- *A misapplication of promotional funding.* Using too much of your budget for ideas, creativity, and production leaves little behind to actually disseminate your message through paid advertising.
- *Not using the materials you produce.* It's common to find perfectly serviceable brochures or patient pamphlets sitting in storage not being used. We're long past the era of being wasteful like this.
- *Not trying new things.* Marketing doesn't involve much science, but it ***is*** experimental. You should be constantly trying new approaches and discarding things that do not work.
- *Not learning from mistakes.* Even after many decades in the business, I'm still making plenty of misjudgments about what might work in a given market or practice setting. Be as intrigued by what doesn't work as you are by what does. Keep asking, "Why?"

• • •

What About Selling?

Selling is a vital subset of medical marketing, but it has an undeservedly bad reputation.

Selling probably first got a bad rap in medicine ages ago, when it was a lot harder to make an accurate diagnosis, much less prescribe an effective cure. But even today, in a field like ophthalmology where we predictably—and lest we forget, almost miraculously—help almost every patient, we do not like to say, "Sell."

"Selling"—the word itself—is much maligned in medicine. Many in ophthalmology are uncomfortable with the notion of selling, seeing it as perhaps coercive, deceiving, and against the patient's best interests.

But we are doing it—this selling—all of the time. Every member of your practice is always selling, mostly unconsciously.

- You are "selling" a job candidate on the benefit of joining your practice rather than a competitor's.
- You are "selling" your landlord on the wisdom of granting concessions in the next lease.
- Your head technician is "selling" their staffer on staying late for patients today.
- Your receptionist is "selling" a caller on making a first appointment.
- Your tech is "selling" the patient on cooperating during the work-up.
- Your glaucoma subspecialist is "selling" their patient in Room 3 on the importance of eye drops.
- And your cataract surgeon in Room 4 is "selling" their patient on the potential benefits of surgery.

From an unabashedly practical business perspective, the chief difference between good and great practices can be boiled down to little more than how well they sell.

- On average, about 15% of North American cataract patients select a PIOL. In some practices, that figure is 25%. What's the difference? *Selling.*
- In the typical general/geriatric practice, about 10% of patients will buy two pairs of glasses during the same shopping trip. In some practices, that figure is 20%. What's the difference? *Selling.*
- In the average practice, a significant percentage of patients push back when the time comes to pay for their modest average refraction fee of about $45. In some practices, however, the refraction fee is $90 or higher, and patients pay without incident. What's the difference? *Selling.*
- The typical no-show rate in America is 5% in an adult ophthalmology practice. But some practices manage a 3% rate. What's the difference? *Selling.*

How well does your practice sell? As an administrator, you can give your staff (and physicians and job applicants) this simple selling skills test.

Hand the person any common object on your desk—it might be a pen, a stapler, or a yellow pad. Then say, "Sell me this."

Excellent sellers—whether they are naturals or formally trained—will rarely hesitate and are generally playful. Just before they start trying to sell your stapler back to you, they will break into a grin.

People with well-developed sales skills will start asking you questions like, "Do you ever have two or more pieces of paper that you would like to permanently clip together, and a temporary paper clip just won't do?" Great salespersons, even during this mock demonstration, won't give up easily—they will persevere, coming at you from different angles, until you are both sharing a laugh over this fun game.

In contrast, poor sellers will first give you a puzzled or anguished look. They do not like this game. Sometimes they'll actually try to bow out, saying, "I'm not very good at this." If you insist on playing, they'll flatly drive to a close, "Would you like to buy this stapler?"—without taking the time to ask about your needs.

You and your people can do better than this. Great selling strides can be made with just a little bit of consciousness raising and by following a few salesmanship pearls. At your next all-hands staff meeting consider using what follows as the start of a formal sales training syllabus.

Effective Selling Pearls in an Ophthalmic Context

- You cannot ethically or effectively sell solutions unless you understand the patient's problems, priorities, and perspectives. You may have witnessed the surgeon who is so cataract-focused that within 30 seconds of seeing a patient with a chief complaint of dry eyes they are recommending cataract surgery. Always address and start solving the ***patient's*** chief complaint first, even if you know that other important eye health conditions are present.
- Have clear, objective, deadline-linked sales objectives. Your goal for enhancing your PIOL practice should not just be expressed as, "More, and as soon as possible"; but something along the lines of, "We would like to increase our PIOL implant rate from 7% to 15% of total cases by the end of this year."
- Remember to address everyone in the exam room and try to understand who the decision maker is going to be. Speak to both the patient and the family member. Ask mom and daughter the questions most relevant to their concerns. Address their respective concerns separately and patiently.
- Try to discriminate between the emotionally based vs the fact-based decision maker. Fact-based patients want to know about how many cases you have performed, your typical outcomes, and the percent of patients who are satisfied with their results. They want to know whether your surgical approach is in the mainstream or is vanguard. Emotional decision makers are more likely to want to know about how the surgery experience is going to go and how it's going to feel to be able to potentially read without glasses for the first time in 25 years.
- Let's say you are a cataract surgeon. After orienting a patient to the treatment options, offer two clear choices rather than one diffuse question like, "So, what do you think?" Instead, ask, "After hearing the two options available, what choice would you prefer, the standard government lens or the advanced technology lens?"
- Salespersons in an earlier era were admonished to "Sell the sizzle, not the steak." Perhaps it's a bit more seemly to say, in the more genteel ophthalmic context, "Let's focus more on the benefits and less on the dry features." More patients are motivated by a description of expected outcomes than by a description of your newest technology.
- Do not fear rejection. Ophthalmologists (and by extension their staff) are conditioned to having patients mostly say, "Yes." Most surgeons hate rejection or even a few reasonable questions. If you are going to effectively provide vanguard or elective care at premium self-pay pricing, you have to be ready to accept a bit more rejection.

Of Office Facilities

Any of you with access to the seashore when you were a child were no doubt fascinated by the hermit crab—that enterprising crustacean who, rather than making its own shell, dons the cast-offs of others in its tide pool.

When the shell its wearing gets a little too pinched, all that Mr. Crab has to do is crawl out of the current premises and stroll naked to the next, larger shell and climb in. No architects to engage. No permits to pull. No wrangling with the general contractor. No cost overruns. No construction defect lawsuits to file.

If only facility development was so easy and cost-free in ophthalmology. Instead, surgeons and their management teams typically undertake much labor and hand-wringing to add even an extra exam lane.

This is an especially vexing process in the current environment, with both headwinds and tailwinds, as the screws of health reform slowly turn, fees fall, patient demands rise, and the ambitions of the most entrepreneurial physicians grow.

To sort it all out, here is a list of a few basic points to ensure that your facility development efforts are in lock-step with your wider business development goals.

- Know your facility utilization numbers. The best, coarse gauge of whether you need more space or not is to count up the number of active, fully equipped exam rooms; multiply by 173 (the nominal number of hours your clinic is open each month); and divide the resulting figure into the number of patients seen in the average month. The resulting figure should be about 1.0, with units of "patient visits per exam room hour." Here's an example:
    - Your practice has five exam rooms.
    - So, you have 5 x 173 = 865 room hours per month.
    - You serve 800 visits per month.
    - Divide 800 visits by 865 room hours, to get 0.9 *patient visits per exam room hour.*

  If your practice has these statistics, your facility is running at only about 90% of potential capacity and you do not need added space. This is obviously a gross, first-pass calculation. Depending on your subspecialty, the availability of optical or special testing space, pace of growth or general layout flaws, and how many peaks and valleys there are in your schedule, you may still be needing more space.
- Explore a "temporal" expansion before adding facilities—that's to say, think about expanding office ***hours*** rather than adding facility ***space*** and cost. If you are trying to make just four exam rooms stretch to serve two doctors who both want to work in "prime time" Monday through Thursday from 9 AM to 4 PM, shift clinic hours around so that the providers are a little less bunched up—one doctor working on Friday in alternate weeks, and running from 8 AM to 5 PM, for example.
- Let's say you absolutely need to expand, but have to do so on a budget:
    - If your budget is tight, eliminate nonessentials. Are you so shy that you really need a private washroom for every doctor? (Over the course of an average year, this owner perk may cost you up to $5 per bathroom break.)

  - The same goes for private doctor office space. (A group office with a meeting table and separate cubicles not only costs less but facilitates communication.)
  - Use cubicles for business staff rather than erecting fixed walls.
  - Fit out a "wow" waiting/reception area, but leave the back clinical space more industrial.
  - Leave out the crown molding, premium carpet, custom wall treatments, and original artwork.
  - Make sure your builder takes a second pass through your architect's plans to "value engineer" the final project.
  - Do not underbuild—if you build for today's needs in a growing practice, the second phase of near-term construction will be far more costly per square foot than being right-sized the first time around.
  - Unless you feel you must, and are very concerned with aesthetics, do not try to win architectural awards with off-beat, expensive designs. Build a box and leave out the curves, both on the shell and on the interior build-out of the practice.
  - Do not buy or build more than you need, but leave room for any obvious, future expansion. Very few ophthalmologists should take the entrepreneurial approach of building the 10,000 square feet they need today, plus another 30,000 square feet to rent to other users.
  - In most cases, create a new facility from the ground up rather than redesigning an existing structure.
  - Do not try to save money by buying cheap, out-of-the-way land … the appreciation of your facility in the coming years will be far lower, ***and*** you'll lose the promotional value of being on a major thoroughfare.
  - If you're in a solo practice and have no solid succession plan, do not build a new facility if you plan to work for fewer than 10 more years. (And if you plan to practice for 10 years or longer, try not to rent, unless you work in a high-priced, inner city environment.)
- Do not overlook exterior appeal. Your senior patients may be avid gardeners. They will "tsk-tsk" your dying shrubbery and assume that your landscaping reflects the quality of your medical and surgical care. Keep up the parking lot's resurfacing and stripes. Purchase the largest/brightest signage local zoning will allow.
- Do not pursue any significant expansion or building project without first preparing a realistic *pro forma* showing the cost-benefit of the project in the years ahead. There are many factors to consider here:
  - Will your total facility costs, as a percent of total collections, be at or under 10% immediately after the project and fall to 6% or less within 5 years?
  - Are you realistic in your projections of how fast practice collections will grow with a new facility?
  - Do you possess the risk tolerance to handle the prospect of having facility costs escalate as a percent of collections if health reform leads to materially lower professional fees?

- What will be the future appreciation on your new property? Will you be able to find a buyer when the time comes or is your area overbuilt with professional space?
- Are you properly hedged and able to carry higher facility costs in the event of a temporary disability, loss of a key provider, or similar difficulty?
- Will your personal net worth be higher or lower in 10 to 20 years if you develop a new facility?

CHAPTER 7

Compatibility and Collaboration With Others

Nature is often hidden, sometimes overcome, seldom extinguished.
—Sir Francis Bacon

Of Adding Value to Patient Relationships

There are two potential responses (both institutionally and personally) to the more difficult environment we find ourselves in today in health care. We can all quietly worry and acquiesce to the fact that each passing year we'll have fewer resources to upgrade provider skills, office amenities, staff training, and surgeon lifestyle.

Or, we can dig deep, apply gumption, and make real organizational progress against the health reform headwinds.

Pinto JB. *Simple: The Inner Game of Ophthalmic Practice Success, Second Edition* (pp 129-151).

If you fall in this second camp, one core driver of success is to add value to our relationship with each patient. Let's examine this more closely. Imagine two doctors, Dr. Success and Dr. Failure. They are each 48 years old and practice in the same urban market.

Dr. Success has about 15,000 active patient charts. He sees these patients on average every 18 months, because he has a sparkling personality—he's the kind of doctor most patients look forward to seeing again for the next visit. His practice has a great recall system and staff who know how to keep patients from slipping away. Patients are always reminded of their appointments, so the no-show rate is low. Those few lost patients who fail to show up are called immediately and shepherded back into the fold.

Dr. Success is versatile. Although he wasn't subspecialty trained, he's competent and stays current, and he's not shy about managing borderline patients that others would typically refer to subspecialists. He also dispenses optical goods, and he has a stake in a local surgery center. As result, his average revenue yield per patient visit is $185. Because he keeps his health up, Dr. Success is energetic and can see about 55 patients a day with energy to spare. In fact, he's so energetic and so loves his work that he only takes 3 weeks off a year. He operates 1 day a week and has 4 full days of clinic.

As you can see, Dr. Success has it all in the relationship and value departments. He has lots of relationships, these relationships are well cemented, and he exchanges a lot of value for a lot of income. His practice revenue is high: about $1.9 million a year. Dr. Success believes in sharing his success, so he pays his competent staff well; therefore, their motivation is high and they help to perpetuate his success. Even so, Dr. Success has a 40% profit margin and has a pretax income of about $760,000 a year, three times above national averages.

By contrast, Dr. Failure, who has been in practice just as long as Dr. Success, has only about 7000 active patient charts, because he's not all that good at developing and maintaining relationships. Dr. Failure sees these patients on average only about every 24 months. His personality is anything but sparkling. In fact, although he was originally trained as well as Dr. Success, Dr. Failure comes across as uncertain when speaking to patients—and this uncertainty is perceived as disinterest... or worse, incompetence.

His practice recall system is almost nonexistent. Dr. Failure figures if patients aren't smart enough to remember to come back in 1 or 2 years, there's no point nagging them—they deserve to get lost. Patients are sometimes reminded of their appointments, but the routing sheets of patients who fail to show up are just tossed out. Dr. Failure loves medical meetings because they're such a great break from the drudgery and stress of practice. But Dr. Failure rarely attends lectures or even networks with his peers. He figures that with his hard job he deserves to sleep in once in a while, hang by the pool, and go shopping.

Dr. Failure may be a little lazy, but at least he's clinically ethical. As his professional skills have eroded year by year, he's freely delegated subspecialty care that is increasingly beyond his grasp. He doesn't dispense glasses, and he's never been invited to be a surgery center partner because his case volumes are simply too low. As result of all this, Dr. Failure's average revenue yield per patient visit is only $135. Dr. Failure is somewhat less than energetic, as you can gather. So, he runs out of gas whenever he has to see more than 30 patients a day, although his average is about 25. Any more than a couple of work-in patients leaves him glaring at his beleaguered appointment clerk.

He works just 4 days a week, and doesn't even come back to the office after his handful of surgical cases every other Wednesday. The combination of not particularly enjoying his practice and being so exhausted at it means that Dr. Failure takes 8 weeks off a year, sometimes more.

As you can see, Dr. Failure is in real trouble. He has relatively few patient relationships after all these years in practice, these relationships are poor, and he exchanges small value for small reimbursements. His practice revenue is only about $475,000 a year. Dr. Failure can barely afford his own salary, much less his staff, so he keeps his skeleton crew low paid and overtaxed, which reinforces their poor interaction with patients. By keeping other costs trimmed, Dr. Failure ekes out a 35% profit margin and has a pretax income of about $166,000 a year, two-thirds of the national average, and only about a fifth of Dr. Success' income.

• • •

There are hundreds of ways to establish and maintain more and better patient relationships, and hundreds more ways of adding value—hundreds of ways to become a "Dr. Success." Sometimes it's hard to see this abstractly by thinking all at once about the multitude of patients you serve. Think, instead, about just a single, typical patient, "Ms. Davis." Someone you saw yesterday. And ask yourself the following:

- Did Ms. Davis have a uniformly pleasant experience when she set up her first appointment? Did she receive a follow-up note welcoming her to the practice and telling her about the practice's policies and scope of services?
- Was the patient or colleague who referred Ms. Davis to your care properly thanked for the referral?
- Did you call Ms. Davis in advance of her appointment? Did you ask her if she had any questions about directions, bringing her medications, or allowing enough time for a complete exam?
- Did the front desk treat Ms. Davis like an old, returning friend? Or an inconvenience, another number to process?
- Was she helped patiently with any paperwork and seen within 20 minutes of her appointment time?
- Did the tech who started Ms. Davis' exam march many steps ahead while escorting her down the hall to Room 2, or did she walk by her side, aiding her if necessary, and enjoying a moment of small talk?
- Did staff refer to Ms. Davis by her proper name unless she insisted otherwise?
- Did you really address Ms. Davis' chief complaint or gloss over this to get to the cataract surgery that you thought was most important?
- Did you look Ms. Davis directly in the eyes (and not just with your slit lamp) when you spoke to her about her chief complaint? Did you touch her appropriately (a pat on the hand or shoulder providing reassurance)? Compliment her on her sharp mind or snappy attire?
- Was Ms. Davis told, "A little stick here," or similar words before her injection, or did you just jab her without warning?
- If she was brave, or even if she wasn't, did you tell her, "Good job?"
- Does Ms. Davis understand what comes next in her treatment plan?

- Does she understand the importance of keeping her next appointment?
- Was Ms. Davis gently and appropriately exposed to other services that you provide? Or did you just assume from her appearance that she was on a fixed income and could never afford new glasses or Botox injections?
- Did you ask Ms. Davis to be sure to refer her friends to the practice? Did you give her cards or brochures to make this easier to do?
- Were her charges explained at checkout? Was a tech tracked down to help answer any last-minute questions?
- Did someone at the checkout desk wish her good day by name? Were they at least the third or fourth person to thank her for coming in that day?
- If Ms. Davis was given a test that will require subsequent interpretation and report writing, will you keep her in the loop promptly on her results?
- If she was a particularly worried patient, will Ms. Davis get a reassuring call from your staff in a few days just to check to see how things are going?
- If she bought glasses, will she get a call in a few weeks to see if they're still comfortable or need adjusting?

Finally, by the end of her exam, was Ms. Davis's relationship with you—and your relationship with her—stronger than when you started? Perfect! That's the surest measure of value exchanged.

• • •

Will it get harder and harder to do all of this in the future? Emphatically yes. Patient expectations are rising just as your resources—and especially the emotional resources needed to be so *darned* nice for so *much less reimbursement* at every encounter—are diminishing. But fortunately, most of the attributes needed to improve the value exchange in a service relationship do not cost a dime. Your same staff who are surly to patients now can learn to be sweet for free if you provide a positive role model and reinforcement, paired with stiff consequences for continued poor patient service.

None of us involved in this wonderful profession of eye care—whether we're surgeons or surgical supporters—like change. But we have to learn how to ride down the road in alignment with the way the traffic is flowing or risk getting run over. Our most worthy competitors are certainly going with the flow and sharpening their relationships … increasing the value they convey to patients at every visit. Their cash flow will show the results. Do not be like Herman in the small story I'll end this with …

> Senior citizen Herman was driving down the freeway. His cell phone rang. "Herman, Herman! Are you OK?!?" says Herman's wife through the phone with a sound of concern. "Of course, Millie," Herman says. "Thank goodness," his wife replies. "I was just listening to the news on the radio. There's a car going the wrong way on the interstate." "It's worse than that," Herman replies. "It's not just one car, it's hundreds of them!!"

Of Working With Family Members in Your Practice

Although no official study has been done, an unofficial check of my files indicates that in something like 10% of all ophthalmic practices, family members are working with each other.

Or perhaps it only seems that way, because a disproportionate number of family-based practices have problems that need outside intercession.

Family based practices come in four basic flavors:

1. Wives or husbands who help their doctor-spouses launch a practice, and then stay on—sometimes longer than originally intended
2. Brothers and sisters who practice with each other (as doctor-partners, or with one sibling as the doctor and one as the administrator)
3. Children of physician-owners who come home to practice medicine or be an office worker with one or both parents
4. Siblings and children of lay office workers who are conveniently tapped as a labor pool

Most of the time, hiring or partnering with family members is a long-contemplated event. You know when your spouse is in their residency that you'll help them launch a practice. You know that your child will be coming in to run the practice after they complete their MBA. But even when you plan well in advance to work with a family member, special problems will crop up that would not be the case when hiring a stranger.

Here are a few guidelines to help you avoid or extract yourself from the most common difficulties.

- *Rule 1: Do not hire anyone you are not willing to fire.* If you are the physician who is hiring a family member, this rule is easy to say—and even discuss and agree to at the outset. The theory is sensible. But execution is tough. Make sure you really mean it before you make the hire. Remember: The average tenure for a new worker (even a doctor) entering your practice is about 4 years (even if some stay for decades). When staff leave you and your practice, it's usually for the better for both parties. Do not block the exit.
- *Abundant meetings, disclosure, and communication are keystones to harmony in a family business.* The need for communication rises materially in family businesses of every type. In some rare cases, this great communication has been present from the outset. More often, teaching family members how to communicate more effectively is at the core of turning around discordant relationships within the practice setting. Go overboard in being transparent with data, meeting minutes, policies, and the basis for making decisions.

- *Get your story straight for nonfamily members.* Job candidates—and particularly doctor and administrator candidates—can be justifiably leery of joining your cozy family practice. Will the nonfamily member be treated as an equal, or will the founder's son, daughter, or spouse be effectively an "untouchable?" In the case of a partner-track associate physician joining a solo practice where the founder's spouse is the administrator, be clear about whether the new doctor will eventually have veto power over who will be the practice's administrator—and how this control will be exercised without undue hurt feelings.
- *The past can be a prelude.* Sibling rivalries can be enduring. I'm often called on to help resolve intrafamily business rivalries. When I take the history from every involved family member within a practice, it is amazing to learn how the current discord has its roots in earlier family dynamics. Struggles for control and leadership, or a parent's affections, can resonate through the years.
- *The business comes first, people second.* This may sound a bit cold, but think of it this way: your practice is a professional workshop as well as an economic engine supporting many other families besides your own. This engine can be harmed, sometimes mortally, when you make the wrong hiring decision. When you begin to suspect you have made the wrong hiring decision, do not focus solely on the hurt feelings of the family member you may need to pull out of the company ... think also, and I would assert primarily, about the interests of the wider company.
- *Arrange a trial hire if possible.* If you're on the fence about having a family member join your practice, try to arrange a readily reversible period of trial employment. Be sure to listen carefully to your staff when they tell you, "We love your (sister, aunt, wife, daughter), but please don't let her work here full time."
- *Consider stopping short of formal employment.* The most common familial addition to a practice is still the spouse-as-administrator. If this is causing difficulties, ask yourself if it would be better for your practice (and your personal relationship with your spouse) to have your spouse take on a more limited role. I've seen numerous cases where a spouse who was ill-suited to be the in-office administrator did a splendid job after shifting to work outside of the clinic as a bookkeeper or marketing coordinator.
- *Get outside help.* Chances are, if you presently work in a family-based practice, you have already been using your attorney, accountant, and various other advisors as referees. This is very healthy, and it can stave off the after-hours frictions that can understandably still smolder when the ophthalmologist has to override a spouse or child working in the office. If you are a physician whose spouse runs the office, urge your spouse to seek external validation before springing a potentially unpleasant (but necessary) change on staff.

- *Familial practice problems can crop up suddenly.* Here is a common scenario. Two ophthalmologists are equal partners. One surgeon's child goes to medical school and, you know what's coming next, in a few years there's a new partner-to-be knocking on the door, full of a sense of entitlement. In principle, the admission of a new partner-track associate should not be colored by family connections. In the real world, wise doctors whose children commence a path to become an eye surgeon will start "what if" discussions early on with their present colleagues.
- *Demonstrate your neutrality.* Unless you are working in the smallest mom and pop practice setting, you must avoid both the appearance and reality of favoritism. Do not let your newly minted doctor-daughter pull rank on your peer partners. Tell her, "Every doctor here had to pay the dues. I love you, but you're going to have to wait your turn like everyone else." Be sure to explain to younger family members joining you in practice that they will have to do twice as much work, twice as well as others, to get half the credit.
- *Do not be afraid to make your practice different.* Although equality is the norm in most group practices, it does not have to be in your setting. If you're the "Papa Doc," and want your son and daughter to take over for you one day, there is nothing wrong with hiring every other provider on terms spelling out that they will be durable associates with no control over operations. The key is disclosure of the special conditions and boundaries from the outset, and then their consistent application.

Of Optometrist Associates

If you're like the typical general ophthalmologist reading this book, you'll see 100 to 200 patients in clinic this week. Unless you're very old school, chances are you could delegate about a third or more of these patients to an optometrist working on your staff.

In America today we have roughly two-and-a-half times as many ODs and MDs/DOs—which suggests that if a two-surgeon practice was aiming at having a full-service eye care center, it would reasonably employ about five optometrists.

A bit more than half of the client practices I serve now employ optometrists, though almost none at a 2.5:1 ratio. Employing ODs is up sharply from a generation ago when only the busiest, and most liberally minded surgeons, were willing to work alongside ODs. If your practice has more patients than professional capacity, you might consider upping optometric staffing ratios to ease the crunch, especially since it's getting much harder and more expensive to hire ophthalmologists.

There are both advantages and disadvantages to hiring an optometrist instead of a fellow ophthalmologist. These are summarized in the following table:

Optometrist	Ophthalmologist
Fairly easily recruited; expect a 2- to 6-month recruitment cycle	Can be extremely difficult to recruit quality individuals, especially in recent years; expect a 1-year or longer recruitment cycle
Lower base salaries, in the range of $80,000 to $120,000 to start for higher-level doctors	Higher base salaries in the range of $150,000 to $300,000+
Generally much lower income-generating capacity and some payer panel access limitations; practice profit augmentation comes not only from direct revenue but from freeing surgeons to take on more secondary and tertiary patients	Potentially much greater ability to generate direct income for the practice and to help support an ancillary ASC
Potentially significant source of revenue from optical dispensing, if allowed to develop their own primary care practice	Limited optical sales augmentation in most cases
Limited succession planning ability; an optometrist can only take over a subset of a retiring surgeon's practice	A professional succession event is relatively easy and seamless
In most state jurisdictions, optometrists can only be business partners with physicians through a labyrinth of shell organizations, although this is liberalizing	Physicians can readily partner with other physicians, facilitating institutional growth and development plans
Even highly skilled ODs are generally content being permanent associates, rather than being partners in the practice; this can be important for surgeon-owners who would prefer to not dilute their ownership position or who desire passive profits	Most ophthalmologist candidates desire and expect partnership positions, which leads to inevitable issues of profit and control dilution for existing partners; it is much harder to build an organization generating passive income for the founders
Professional boundaries, authority, and reporting lines are generally clear; optometrists readily defer medical and management decisions to MD-owners	Struggles for authority and autonomy by junior doctors are far more common; in the best of settings, this results in a stronger organization, but it can also reduce practice harmony

The first step before you start placing ads is to clarify the scope of work actually needed in your practice. Optometrists can fill several different, sometimes overlapping roles. Here are the most common:

- *Refractionist or super-tech.* A few surgeons use optometrists as refractionists only. This is a vast underutilization of resources. In the most efficient practices, technicians (and technology) do the refracting and patients just have to see one doctor during a visit—an optometrist or ophthalmologist—based on their needs.

- *Clinical support staffing director.* Once a practice has more than three or four technicians, it's wise to select a supervisor for this group. In the absence of an appropriate lay staffer for this important job, an optometrist can be a fine choice. Optometrists will typically do this supervisory work on top of a full or nearly full clinic schedule.
- *Technician training director.* Optometrists often have more time and patience to elevate technical staffing competency and can add real value as the practice's resident "professor."
- *Co-management center director.* Practices dependent on optometric referrals are often concerned that adding an optometrist to the staff will kill referrals. The reverse is actually the case. The most successful co-management centers have learned that hiring an optometrist as a manager or senior director of the practice (with duties split between outreach and direct patient care) actually stimulates community referrals.
- *Separate/autonomous practitioner within your practice.* Practices with a diversified service base that includes dispensing and primary care should be delegating all appropriate patients to an optometric provider, rather than tying up surgeon time. In such settings, you should have formal, written care pathways specifying which patients—new and returning—go where. Most surgeons find that optometric practice autonomy works best when accompanied by periodic, grand-rounds style reciprocal chart reviews so ODs and MDs within the same practice are applying the same standard of care.
- *Chief or "homeroom" clinician in a satellite office.* A hub-and-spoke practice, with one core office and numerous satellites, can be an extremely viable business model. I've found through the years that the most important success factors include having a resident doctor who is in the practice daily for both patient and staff continuity. An optometrist can fill this role at low cost and with great loyalty to the home office.

• • •

Hiring a new optometrist (or properly managing the doctors you have) should start with a position description. This should include the following elements:

- *Scope of practice.* The practice's optometrists will practice to the highest levels permitted by state practice regulations and payer stipulations, and within the boundaries set by the medical director.
- *Supervision.* Optometrists will report to the medical director of the practice (or can report to the optometric director, a chief OD selected in larger practices, who in turn reports to the medical director).
- *Practice volume.* The practice optometrist will see a mix of postoperative patients, routine patients, and treatment follow-up cases. Depending on patient mix, the optometrist is expected to see between 22 and 35 patients per day with two exam rooms, a dedicated technician, and float staff who will be available to step in at higher volumes.

- *Location of practice.* The practice's optometrists, like all professional staff, may be called upon to see patients in various locations throughout our service region and have the flexibility to occasionally provide care in less-than-optimal settings.
- *Days and hours worked.* Full-time optometrists are expected to work not less than 40 hours per week and may be called upon to work additional hours to fulfill all professional duties. To optimize use of the practice's office facilities, optometrists may be required to conduct early morning, evening, and weekend clinics.
- *Practice emergency call.* Subject to hospital regulations, community standards, and practice policy, practice optometrists share call or first call with ophthalmologists.
- *Staff education.* Optometrists share with the practice's surgeons in staff education duties.
- *Meetings and assistance with management projects.* Optometrists participate on various practice management committees and may be called on to lead various initiatives and projects for the practice.
- *Community service and promotion.* All professional staff are expected to give no fewer than three talks in the community per year, which will be scheduled by the practice administrator. Staff optometrists are strongly urged, especially in their initial years getting established, to join a community service organization, such as Lions, Rotary, etc.
- *Outreach to fellow optometrists.* If the practice seeks optometric referrals from providers in the community, staff optometrists may be called upon to help in this area.

• • •

As with eye surgeons, not all optometrists are created equally. As a broad generalization, younger ODs, and especially those with residency training, are better prepared to step into a busy ophthalmic practice. Sparkly doctors, both in intelligence and energy terms, can see more patients than dull docs. Recruiting a high-quality optometrist is generally much easier than finding a top-flight ophthalmologist. Journal ads and letters to doctors in the state or region will almost always yield an acceptable candidate in short order. It pays to aim for a higher-quality doctor; small increments in compensation can yield large benefits in productivity and ease of management.

Once your new doctor is on board, use the sample position description outlined previously to set and manage to highly specific performance standards. When I'm called on to untangle OD performance snarls, the first thing I address are the basics of the practice's written expectations for the doctor. More often than not, when there's a problem such documents are absent. In addition, ongoing management of your practice's optometrists should include their attendance at all-hands doctor meetings at least once a month. Nothing can reduce optometric morale and performance faster than being left out of meetings and feeling professionally marginalized.

As for the future, optometric training is improving, as is the average quality of students entering optometry school. Legalistically, the optometric scope of practice is widening and optometrists will increasingly be allowed to partner with MDs and DOs. Close, collaborative, economically integrated practice between the "O's" will sooner rather than later be the norm.

Of Meetings

Meetings are simultaneously the worst and most important part of any effort to run a better eye care organization, "worst" because few managers and physicians truly relish them, and "important" because no practice with two or more people can survive without them.

In the scores of practice performance audits I conduct each year, there is a direct correlation between the quality, frequency, and duration of meetings and the profitability of each reviewed practice. Indeed, some the most successful practices consciously cannibalize productive clinical hours each month to find sufficient meeting time.

Here are 10 pearls on how to get the best results in the least meeting time:

1. Have a set calendar of meetings made up at least a quarter in advance. It's best to hold most meetings midweek, with enough time at the start of the week to plan and enough time left in the week to execute. Post this calendar prominently, and do not tolerate staff or doctors who chronically miss meetings or are tardy. Consider a fine for absent doctors.
2. Periodically combine doctors and managers in group meetings, rather than having each half of the practice meet separately. Arrange an "executive committee" style of management, where the practice's MP, administrator, and managers from every department meet every couple of weeks to interpret and apply board policy and organize the nuts and bolts of the practice. In the best practices, and almost universally in very large ones, department heads participating with such meetings are given details of the practice's finances and are responsible for a departmental budget—they should be ***profit*** managers, not just ***process*** managers.
3. Avoid the error of too many practice board participants. If your practice has more than 12 to 15 owners, streamline your physician board to an elected subset of owners on the board, converting to representational governance.
4. In smaller practices, especially those still run by the consensus of all partners rather than formal votes, board meetings tend to be relatively informal. These should be held at least monthly and concentrate on setting policy and covering the high points of operations oversight, rather than micromanagement. Shift to the formality of motions and votes if your discussions are bogging down.
5. In large practices, standing committees (eg, marketing, clinical affairs, compensation, finance) can reduce larger meetings to quarterly events. Such committees need not be more than two people in some cases. Avoid the temptation to be overly democratic by having too many subcommittees and every staff member serving on a committee. Do not create standing committees when a single individual or a brief, focused task force effort will do.
6. Depending on the scope and pace of change in your practice and your geographic coverage, all-hands staff meetings should be held anywhere from monthly to annually. Whatever the intervals, these should have a tightly scripted agenda and be largely upbeat events. You'll know you're doing it right when department managers and staff are speaking for more than half of the meeting time. You'll know you're doing it wrong when the administrator and physicians spend the entire meeting giving speeches.

7. Each supervisor should be responsible for calling and running their own department's meetings. In too many practices, such meetings are a command performance held for the doctors' or administrator's benefit. Because few department supervisors are professionally trained as managers, they should receive ongoing mentoring on how to run effective meetings. The MP and the administrator should periodically attend each department's meeting.
8. Here are tips for the smallest meetings in your practice. Individual staff should have their performance evaluated by their supervisors at least annually—twice a year is preferred, as well as at the end of any probationary period. Disciplinary and termination meetings should be held at the end of the workday or week, and in most cases should include a witness. Exit interviews with staff who are voluntarily separating should sometimes be as long and detailed as pre-employment interviews, to find out why a member of your staff is leaving and how the practice can do better next time.
9. Remember that meetings are meaningless without follow-up action on agreed tasks. Make sure that the minutes you keep include a system for setting and tracking deadlines and the person responsible for each agreed project.
10. A strong practice manager is no substitute for physician involvement with all of these meetings. In fact, the strongest managers demand doctor participation. The frequency of meetings in the best-run practices will continue to increase in step with the increasing complexity of new regulations, higher standards for providing quality care, decreasing reimbursement, and increasing competition.

Of Conflicts

When you work with others in a practice, even with colleagues you otherwise like and admire a great deal, the easiest and most human thing to slip into is a conflict. The hardest thing—at least in some practice settings—is to resolve the conflict and restore good relationships. As has been said of marriage, partnering involves expectations and expectations (without lots of communication to adjust them and make them more reasonable) beget conflict.

Conflict, whether between nations, condo neighbors, or eye surgeons, is a side effect of proximity. Partnerships undergo conflict in only two situations: when the business is doing quite well and when it is doing poorly. Which is to say that all practices undergo conflict to one degree or another pretty much all of the time. As C.T. Lawrence Butler, an author on conflict resolution, puts it, "Peace is not the absence of conflict, but rather the ability to resolve conflict without violence."

The most harmonious practices are superior to the extent that they actively preempt conflict through better/clearer rules and communication and manage conflict formally and in a conscientious, stepwise fashion when it occasionally arises.

In my travels throughout the country, practice conflicts are at their most acrimonious level where the basics of communication and governance are absent:

- Leadership boundaries and reporting lines are unclear; there may be a figurehead doctor-leader, but not a formal MP who has a formal position description and granted authorities.
- Board meetings are infrequent, and when they do occur, they are shallow and brief—substantive, root-of-the-conflict discussions are avoided.
- Performance expectations—if overtly expressed at all—are oral rather than written.
- Rather than following written corporate rules, especially the rule that the majority vote wins in the boardroom, you drive for 100% consensus on every issue, which can be very frustrating to try to achieve.

An important, underlying organizational gap, one that spawns numerous conflicts, is the lack of a written strategic business plan spelling out the future of the company. It's easy to see how conflicts might arise from this. If you haven't formalized growth goals for your practice (eg, the geographic span of the practice, the provider mix, growth targets), how are you going to avoid conflicting views about tactics like opening a satellite, adding a new partner, or buying a new piece of capital equipment?

A central resource needed to both prevent conflicts and tamp them back down when they arise is transparent, well-understood economic statistics. Most business conflicts boil down to money arguments. If you only go over practice finances at the annual meeting or pursue emotional arguments for or against a course of action without consulting the objective financial impact, your conflicts will drag on for months without resolution.

Money conflicts within the practice are, of course, often due to or at least compounded by money conflicts at home. If you're the surgeon of your family, and you and your spouse are at odds because you are not earning enough to cover the family's current expenses, you're going to vote down projects in the boardroom that may be in the practice's and your partner's best interests. As we enter an era of major health care payment reform, which will constrict most incomes, it is critical that all practice owners gain control over their personal living costs to avoid compounding boardroom arguments.

Resolving Conflicts

Even though partner-to-partner conflicts can feel like the interpersonal equivalent of war, we no longer resort to duels for conflict resolution (as satisfying as that would be in some settings!).

Instead, partners have to resort to more genteel alternatives. The conflict resolution efforts you pursue should be progressive. Let's look at an example: discord about the declining surgical skills of the senior ophthalmologist—a conflict that can occasionally surface in group practices.

Here's the setup for the birth of a conflict:

- Dr. Smith is 74; he's the founder and MP of a four-surgeon group practice.
- His next-nearest partner, Dr. Jones, is 68.

- Smith bristled at a recent board meeting when his two youngest partners, Drs. Able and Baker, both in their 40s, gently suggested that he should retire from surgery.
- Jones thinks that Smith's surgical skills are just fine and came to his defense.
- The discussion heated up rapidly, tempers flared, and the board meeting came to a bitter close.

What should happen next? In a setting like this, conflict resolution proceeds through five progressive steps:

1. *Unilateral resolution through acquiescence.* Dr. Smith, the senior surgeon, could resolve the conflict unilaterally. He could simply admit to his junior partners that he, too, has been concerned about his cataract outcomes, and he's ready to limit his practice to medical ophthalmology. On the other side of the argument, Drs. Able and Baker could similarly yield, reconsider their position, apologize to the practice founder, and simply agree to drop the matter for the time being. Coming from one side or the other of a dispute, such acquiescence resolves the conflict briskly, cheaply, and simply.
2. *Internal, unfacilitated resolution.* Let's imagine that neither side is backing down. Once tempers cool, the partners meet again. The facts are examined about Dr. Smith's true outcome statistics. Rational discussion between peers could lead to several, quite satisfactory endpoints. Smith might agree to operate only until the end of the year or to limit his practice to uncomplicated cases. Or, the facts may bear out that Dr. Smith's patient care is completely within contemporary norms. This, along with unilateral acquiescence, is the easiest trajectory of conflict. It's the least costly and time consuming, and the approach most likely to preserve—even strengthen—group harmony.
3. *Facilitated resolution.* When two kids on the playground can't work out their differences, a teacher or principal usually gets involved. The ophthalmic equivalent of this is to call on an agreed-upon internal or external facilitator to untangle the dispute. Such a facilitator is generally an expert on the matter at hand. If partners cannot agree on a staffing issue, they can simply agree to let their administrator, labor lawyer, or department head break the tie. If the partners are stuck on a facility issue, they can turn to a local real estate or architectural expert. In this case regarding Dr. Smith's surgery, the partners could ask a local, neutral colleague to weigh in and agree in advance to abide with the colleague's judgment in the matter.
4. *Alternative dispute resolution.* If the partners are still at an impasse on Dr. Smith's surgical skills, dispute resolution can move up the ladder and get more formal, but still fall short of resorting to bitter and costly legal intervention. Your practice's general legal counsel (ie, whose client is formally your practice entity, not you or its other individual owners) may step in personally to negotiate a partner settlement or guide you to the services of a paid alternative dispute resolution expert—an arbitrator or mediator who can help you stop short of resorting to the legal system.

5. *Formal legal resolution.* "Lawyering up" and battling in the courts is the very last means of dispute resolution you and your partners want to employ. This is the costly, emotionally taxing, and time-consuming end of the line. It's the business equivalent of radical surgery and chemotherapy, from which the "practice-as-patient" may not survive, even if the dispute is resolved.

• • •

Unless you practice alone as a soloist, and can control your professional environment by fiat, you and your colleagues will have to resolve numerous disputes each year. Disputes—like unwarranted patient complaints and surgical complications—simply come with practice ownership.

In the healthiest settings, dispute resolution happens organically and without any holdover rancor. With strong leadership from an administrator and MP, each principal's divergent positions are respected, dignities are preserved, and molehills are not inflated into mountains. When the occasional "really big deal" surfaces that cannot be handled with a bit more boardroom discussion time, the group's leaders push the issue fearlessly through progressively greater levels of formality until a fair and satisfactory outcome is achieved.

Of Physician Bullying

The most fortunate of us with any leanings toward becoming a bully are punched in the snoot by the time we reach the sixth grade and reform our ways. Unfortunately, some nascent bullies are able to avoid a good thrashing. Of these, I'm afraid a few too many become ophthalmologists.

Why do these otherwise talented and admirable people become the worst kind of coward? And what can the rest of us do to deal with them? All too many who work in ophthalmology wrestle with these questions in the workplace.

Hopefully some self-recognition—and self-reform—will be sparked by what follows.

• • •

Why Do People Bully?

According to the British anti-bullying website, www.bullyonline.org, "The purpose of bullying is to hide inadequacy … anyone who chooses to bully is admitting their inadequacy, and the extent to which a person bullies is a measure of their inadequacy." Bullies, it goes on to say, project their inadequacy onto others:

- To avoid facing up to their inadequacy and doing something about it
- To avoid accepting responsibility for their behavior and the effect it has on others
- To reduce their fear of being seen for what they are, namely weak, inadequate, and often incompetent individuals
- To divert attention away from their inadequacy

In ophthalmology, we see bullying behavior at some of the highest levels of the profession—in MPs, department chairs, and highly vetted subspecialists.

The early roots of bullying are easy to understand intuitively as a lay person: abusive family backgrounds, low self-esteem, and a history of having been bullied oneself. Seen through this lens, the typical bully perhaps deserves as much sympathy, even pity, as loathing.

How Ophthalmologists Bully

In 40 years on the road, I've seen it all:

- The surgeon who throws instruments, projecting their own incompetence on innocent scrub techs
- The ophthalmologist who up-ends a staffer's stool in the OR, sending them to the hospital
- The eye doctor who sneers at patients for asking a perfectly reasonable question about their care
- The practice owner who screams at their administrator about adverse business performance—which is in reality driven by the doctor not the manager
- Progressively florid swearing as a substitute for calm, clear communication
- Giving the "silent treatment" and similar power-tripping
- Nitpicking about one technician's alleged failings, while letting the same performance gaps slide for the rest of the crew

The Cost of Bullying

Physicians are smart and self-interested. Those who are bullies commonly justify their behavior because, "My staff won't perform unless I chew on them." Many of the surgeon-bullies I've counseled through the years believe they owe it to their patients to be harsh with staff in order to impose higher standards on patient care. "After all," they say, "that's how I was trained in medical school."

They could not be further from reality in holding this sentiment.

Bullying subordinates actually ***reduces*** their performance and retards workers' willingness to grow and improve their skills. Bullying reduces morale and increases staff turnover, and it creates practice organizations from which the most confident and accomplishing staff flee, leaving behind the least competent workers—those willing, like battered spouses, to stick around because they "obviously deserve to be abused."

The Three Types of Ophthalmologist Bullies

In my experience, surgeon bullies come in three basic varieties:

1. *Episodic/improvable.* In a moment of stress, the surgeon lashes out—uncharacteristically—at others. We are all prone to this in varying degrees, and in the mildest cases the episodic bully rapidly pulls back from the brink, recognizes the pain and harm they have caused in others, and quickly apologizes. Ideally, this kind of bully learns from each outburst and over time improves their behavior. The seriousness of episodic bullying is, of course, in the eye of the beholder. The established surgeon who loses it once or twice a year (or the stressed-out young surgeon who is still trying to get a grip) is pretty easy to forgive and live with.
2. *Chronic/escalating.* This kind of sociopathic surgeon-bully gets worse over time. When fresh staff members first start working with them, the newness and formality of the professional relationship may keep the bully at bay. But over time, the boundaries come down and the bullying behavior escalates, until the new staffer has to wince just as much as the veterans.
3. *Second-hand bullying.* Bullying is largely a learned behavior. Those who are part of a work group led by a bully will commonly start to become bullies themselves.

Responding to Ophthalmologist Bullies

Life was easy (and less litigious) in grammar school, where you could simply stand up to the schoolyard bully, bop them a good one (like your dad may have showed you!), and be done with it. Whether you are the peer-colleague of a bully in your practice, a manager, or a line staffer, if you are the target of bullying you have four basic recourses:

1. You can ***ignore*** the perpetrator. Not reacting to a bully generally stimulates their escalating efforts to control you, but if your practice is large enough and full of alternate victims, you may find it possible to bore your bully into pestering someone else.
2. You can ***confront*** the surgeon-bully. This sometimes works, particularly when the bully is the "episodic/improvable" variety. At the very most, your strong confrontation may be enough of a wake-up call to cease the bully's behavior. At the very least, the bully may leave you alone and pick on a weaker victim.
3. You can ***report*** the bully to a higher authority. This is the best recourse in a larger group practice. Administrators and practice boards understand and want to avoid the high cost of workplace harassment. As the average practice size grows in America, solo and small practices linger on as the last refuge of bully-surgeons who can skirt institutional oversight. Indeed, if you contemplate leaving your current practice to get away from a bullying doctor, consider joining a larger practice.
4. You can ***withdraw*** from the practice. This is the most practical approach and the move most immediately under your control.

What can't you do? You cannot try to elevate the level of your performance and expect that the surgeon-bully will lay off of harassment. If anything, you'll invite more attention by generating even more jealousy and feelings of inadequacy over your terrific performance.

Of Collaboration

Practicing ophthalmology, in today's formidable environment, obliges the juxtaposition of two quite different, and often conflicting, personalities and management styles: the naturally independent style of surgeons and the necessarily collaborative style of business managers.

When faced with a problem, the inclination of most surgeons is to say, "Let ***me*** operate." The manager with a problem is more likely to say, "Let ***us*** call a meeting."

What works best, autonomy or collaboration? Both styles have their place, and both can lead to tremendous problems in your practice when misapplied. A surgeon obviously cannot operate by committee, any more than a manager can act completely autonomously.

But as practices get larger, and both the medical and commercial dimensions of modern practice become more complex, it's important to steer toward more and more collaboration at all levels.

Improved collaboration can be achieved with effort in just four practical areas that we'll call channels, communication, open sharing, and delegation. Let's explore each of these in turn.

Channels

The unfortunate assumption of many staff in the typical ophthalmology practice is that they're to be seen and not heard. As a result, many support staff won't tell you what they think unless they're directly asked. Not much collaboration will happen until you open up channels, and this has to be more than setting up a suggestion box. You won't get great input until you ask for it. Here are some examples of practical, underused channels:

- If you're the administrator or MP of your practice, sit down for coffee or lunch with two or three lay staff at a time to informally talk shop. Spend 90% of your time listening. The channels you open with the first few meetings will make these same staff members more comfortable approaching you when problems or opportunities arise—even before you ask.
- Meet at least quarterly with associate providers. Review their performance statistics and draw them out about their career goals.
- It can be especially useful to open channels with staffers who are about to leave your practice on good terms. Such staff are often willing to be more candid than employees who remain behind about the problems they see.

Communication

This needs to take place at every level of your practice and, with increasing practice scale, needs to steer toward the formality of written rather than oral communication.

- Meetings have always been the bane of medical organizations. But meetings are an irreducible obligation in the best of practices. As a rule of thumb, budget for each week an average of at least 1 hour of doctor time and 90 minutes of nonsupervisory lay staff time spent in meetings. These figures more than double for managers and MPs. If you're spending any less time than this, you are probably not communicating and connecting enough to keep up the pace of collaboration.

- In the typical mid-sized practice, the various job descriptions, policy documents, and procedure manuals should run to hundreds of pages altogether. It's grueling to create the first draft of these reference materials, but much easier to collaborate on procedures and constantly improve them if these are formally written down.
- As a surgeon-owner, even if you have already made a decision, sometimes it's important to ask others for their opinion. This can be done with a few informal hallway conversations, or more formally in a group meeting or written survey.
- In larger practices, when a new policy has been made, it's helpful to post it in writing for a comment period. Let's say you've just decided that half of all staff vacation time should be scheduled during doctor downtime. Even if you're firmly committed to this new policy, giving staff the courtesy of input can take the sting out of it—and you may actually receive suggestions that improve the new policy.

Open Sharing

When I conduct surveys of client staff, their greatest frustration is rarely centered on wages or work conditions—lay staff most commonly complain that they do not get enough feedback and information, especially from practice owners. It's incredibly helpful to let your entire staff know about your future plans for the practice and your reasons behind office priorities and policies. When the going gets tough you do not have to be "Dr. Sunshine" when collaborating in this way. Be candid about difficulties in the practice—the more brains you plug into each problem, the better the solutions will be.

Delegation

Collaboration means sharing. And sharing—in a business context—often means delegation:

- Practice board meetings commonly bog down with minutia. Push decisions as far down the organization chart as you can.
- Doctors should not be making decisions that can be handled by the administrator. Adept administrators don't make decisions than can be handled by department heads.
- When a decision involves more than one practice department, choose staff from each impacted area of your practice to weigh in on the matter.

• • •

One particularly efficient process to foster collaboration is called "nominal group technique" (NGT). In just a few minutes, several staff members or doctors in a group meeting (up to about 20 people) can dissect problems, weigh numerous solutions, and democratically arrive at a consensus. Although there are several variants on NGT, here's a four-step process I think you'll find effective in achieving "groupthink."

1. Choose a moderator and hand out pens and paper to the group. Read a clear statement of the problem at hand. For example: "We have agreed that a complete new patient exam should not take more than 65 minutes. However, based on our latest time study, the average time is 83 minutes and only a third of our patients are checking out within our agreed 65-minute deadline. How can we solve this problem and improve clinic flow?"
2. Announce that everyone has 3 to 5 minutes to privately brainstorm all the possible solutions, writing their ideas down along the way on the paper they have been given (these are not to be handed in).
3. When the minutes are up, call time. Then go around the room and ask every member of the group to describe ***one*** of their solutions. As this is done, no one should comment or shoot down any of the ideas. Go around the room as many times as it takes to get everyone's ideas expressed. As each participant describes his or her ideas, a scribe should write these down (and number each) on a flip chart or white board.
4. It's not unusual to get dozens of possible solutions up on the board. Next, vote as a group on the best ideas. Ask the group to write down the numbers corresponding with the best three solutions on the board. Then go around the room and get everyone's votes—the scribe records these.

If the moderator moves things along briskly, NGT can generate a collaborative, ranked-order list of great solutions to even the toughest problems in under 30 minutes. You can apply the NGT process or a more orthodox, open, group discussion to refine each of your top solutions.

• • •

Groupthink is definitely the way to go. But don't go overboard. It's easy for everyone to fall in line behind the emerging trend of the group, even if that trend is wrong. In the midst of collaboration and teamwork, there is still a vital role for members of a group to speak up and go against the popular tide. Researchers have found that the most effective way to avoid this herd mentality from taking over during group meetings is to make sure that the group is as diverse as possible. To this end, a meeting on the scheduling template should include technicians, receptionists, and managers—not just doctors. A meeting on budgeting for the next year should include not just practice insiders, but the practice's outside finance and accounting counsel.

Of Mergers and Acquisitions

Practice mergers (ie, the economic integration of Practice A and Practice B into a new and larger group) and acquisitions (ie, Practice A buying Practice B, with only Practice A remaining as a legal entity) are fueled by three core incentives: anxiety, avarice, or ambition.

Until recently, practice mergers and acquisitions activity was relatively quiescent, except for in the mid-1990s, when practice consolidation was a mania driven by Wall Street and health reform worries. We are now seeing a resurgence in such transactions. This time around, however, rather than Wall Street we have private equity company transactions surfacing (eg, Varsity Healthcare Partners, Candescent Partners, and more to follow) as well as a proliferation of private, practice-to-practice deals and a trickle of hospital deals.

The incentives are more varied today, and they are not just based in fear. These incentives include:

- Sharing increasingly expensive testing and treatment equipment
- Paying for marketing costs that have risen steeply in recent years
- Providing patients with a deeper team of subspecialists
- Pooling case volumes sufficient to support the development of an ASC or laser center
- Preparing for an anticipated tougher reimbursement environment, where you may have open access to patients (unlike the last era of prepaid health plan development) but be obliged to be markedly more efficient in using fixed-cost resources to thrive
- Responding to the formation of *other* large groups in town
- Health care systems rounding out their employed provider base

Practice-to-practice marriages present at least as many social nuances and intrigues as two single parents merging households, with the added complexities borne of scale, regulatory burden, and financial intricacy.

The long run-up to any merger transaction includes a series of meetings between the principals and senior lay staff of each side. When I moderate these merger conferences, the agenda focuses on the resolution of a few predictable, open issues. I've listed the 17 most important of these issues next—generically in this case. If you're contemplating a merger in your local market, a review of this list may help you decide, even before the first formal meeting, if you're ready to take the next step.

1. Is a merger even the appropriate transaction, or should this deal be something else? An acquisition? A strategic alliance? A purchase option agreement? Or, a narrower partnership to develop a surgery center or shared satellite?

2. What are the drivers for your merger transaction? Here are a few common examples:
    - Succession planning
    - Admiration of the target practice or practitioner
    - Geographic benefits (ie, covering service area gaps in your regional market)
    - Improved contract access
    - Expense sharing (ie, developing a central billing office or combining marketing staff)
    - Cooperative ancillary facility development
    - Supporting, as a group, a retinal or glaucoma subspecialist you can't support on your own
    - Building to a scale allowing effective competition with a dominant practice (ie, the second and third largest practices may merge to eclipse the largest market player)
3. What issues are potentially retarding a transaction? Some retardants include:
    - Excessive near-term transaction or consolidation costs, pushing gains well off into the future
    - Difficulty identifying equal and reciprocal benefits
    - Clinical or business philosophies that differ
    - Interpersonal conflicts between principals or key management staff
    - Simply, the passage of too much time—early interest in an iffy-but-worthy transaction can yield to boredom and then antipathy if pace and momentum are not maintained. Time is generally not a friend of prospective merger transactions.
4. What are the details of the transaction strategic plan? Is there an agreed, common vision? Are the principals aligned and hot to pursue this, or merely lukewarm? What is the desired endpoint practice and how fast will we get there? What is everyone's tolerance for risk or deferment of income? If merging will lead to the purchase of new facilities or costly equipment, is everyone prepared personally to take on debt?
5. Are there other local practices we should consider as subsequent consolidation targets? Your prospective merger may be just the first move in a real-life chess game. If this is the case, do the original merger parties agree on who the subsequent tuck-in targets should be?
6. How long will each provider continue to practice, what will be their retirement trajectory (eg, abrupt or gradual), and are there successors in line to step in?
7. Who is going to be the administrator of the new practice—an existing manager or someone new and neutral? Which staff members will advance in their careers? Which staffers will be redundant and terminated, and how can they be treated most fairly?

8. Are we going to immediately collapse lay staff wage and benefit differentials, phase changes in over time, or grandfather in existing staff? How soon will we change staff policies, uniforms, operational details, training protocols, etc?
9. What will be the name of the converged practice? Will we pursue a repositioning and the creative design work associated with this? How can we leverage the market strengths of each respective party in the new practice?
10. Who will own what after the merger? How will the values of the respective practices (and the equity owned by each constituent partner) be derived? Will the by-doctor ownership of the newly merged practice be equal (ie, each of four partners now owns 25%) or unequal? Will there be proportional or disproportionate ownership in all practice segments (eg, the core practice, ASC, optical, equipment leasing company, real estate entity)?
11. What will be the form of business … a partnership, limited liability company, professional corporation, etc?
12. How will practice governance change? What will be the chain of command and what will the organization chart look like? How often will the board meet? What future conflict resolution procedures will be used? What will be the financial performance reporting intervals? What agreed normative benchmarks will prevail?
13. Will any policies limit the outside business activities of partners (ie, in unaffiliated optical or ASC entities in the market)?
14. Who will be the initial MP or medical director? What will their term of office be? What authorities will be granted? Will the MP be paid a stipend for this important work?
15. What provider compensation methodology will be used initially, and how will this be reviewed from time to time? What about benefits and officer entitlements? What maximum vacation and education time off will be permitted to partners? If excessive time is taken off by a partner, what penalty will this trigger?
16. How and for what offenses can an inappropriate partner be bumped down to associate or removed from the practice? Will founding partners be in a special category and somehow shielded from removal? How will noncompete issues be handled? Will competitive prohibitions be absolute or will we take a liquidated damages approach?
17. Who will remain on the endpoint practice's advisory team: lawyers, accountants, compliance, and various other advisors?

• • •

Merging ophthalmologists is a bit like tying cats together by the tail. It's rough on the cats and not so easy on the cat wranglers, either. Thoughtful answers to these and scores of deeper questions can help to increase the odds of merger and acquisition success. And, perhaps, even reduce the odds of feline distemper.

CHAPTER 8

Partnering

Man prefers to believe what he prefers to be true.
—Sir Francis Bacon

Of Partnership

What is a partner, really? Dictionaries say things like: "A partner is someone involved in a close, cooperating relationship with others, regulated by mutual rights and responsibilities, to further a common enterprise." But this is pretty ice cold.

Partnerships, the good ones, are alive and full of passion. I like this definition better: "A partner is someone with whom you achieve things that would be difficult or impossible to achieve alone."

Pinto JB. *Simple: The Inner Game of Ophthalmic Practice Success, Second Edition* (pp 153-168).

Ophthalmic partnerships fall into two very broad and profoundly different categories:

1. *Unequal partnerships: Surprise!* This is the most common form of partnership, in eye care and elsewhere. Even if partners are legally and economically equal, they are rarely equal in actuality. An examination of the typical ophthalmology practice reveals a rank order of leaders and followers. The hierarchy is most commonly along lines of either tenure (who came first?), economic production (who collects the most?), or natural leadership (who by raw personality is granted the most authority?). In these kinds of partnerships, decisions and resource allocations are lopsided. But so long as everyone agrees to this approach ahead of time, unequal partnerships can work just fine.
2. *Equal partnerships.* In these rare partnerships, doctors generally have equal shares in the practice and all of its subsidiaries such as optical shops, buildings, and surgery facilities. Both younger and older doctor partners have an equal voice in management. Perhaps the most important contribution to harmony is that everyone in an equal partnership setting gets what they deem to be a fair share of resources. Marketing dollars are split fairly among the various subspecialists. Everyone gets to rotate through the most productive satellite offices. Qualified and interested doctors take turns at being the MP. Perhaps most importantly, all partners rise or fall with the total success of the total organization.

• • •

When two or more doctors draw themselves together, the kind of partnership they choose—equal or unequal—has huge implications for everyone around them. In an equal partnership, the practice administrator is less likely to take sides. In equal partnerships, even junior staff realize that it will be hard to play one doctor off the other. I suspect that even patients get a sense that all doctors are interchangeable and are more willing to see whichever doctor is most available. I think the reverse is also true. If there's clearly a dominant, "head" doctor, patients gravitate to that one provider, especially for their surgical care. This can amplify and leverage rivalries that naturally occur in unequal partnerships.

It's more likely for truly mutual, equal partnerships to form naturally when two young, equally novice doctors start a practice together. Equality is far less common when a young surgeon joins an established doctor. In these situations, the young surgeon, even after a successful associateship, will likely remain in the senior doctor's shadow until the older doctor retires.

A discussion of partnership models wouldn't be complete without reviewing how young surgeons make it through the ranks from employed associate to partner.

I've always been critical of the all-or-nothing approach most commonly taken in private practice medical employment, where junior doctors are often moved after 2 or 3 years, in one leap, from "associate" to "full partner." This works against basic human nature and the experience of most large institutions (eg, military, educational, religious, trade union, business, political). These institutions move their members from novice to expert in small, incremental stages. Perhaps in the future we'll decide that the most intelligent approach is to grant similar, incremental shares—"merit badges," if you will—so that junior doctors feel a sense of steady progression in their early years (and are not so overwhelmed by a high initial buy-in cost).

Whether partners are equal or unequal, the biggest predictor of success and harmony is mutual agreement about the development path of the practice. Partnerships are hardest to maintain when there are no large goals held in common. And yet, very few group practices have anything like a written business plan. The angriest doctors I counsel are those with partners who do not share their goals, or far worse, hold them back from accomplishing their dreams.

Finally, some doctors do not really play well in groups, and should probably not be part of a partnership, just as some people should probably not be married. It may take you several years of struggle (or several practice divorces) to learn this about yourself.

Of Adding a New Doctor

Before we confuse ourselves with the details, and in keeping with the theme of this book, it's helpful to remember that for all the complexities and frustrations that come with running an eye clinic, we have only two core dimensions of your practice to manage: your ***volume*** of patients and your ***capacity*** to serve them.

The first, patient volume, is largely controlled with internal and external marketing. The second, capacity, is solved with a checkbook—to buy new facilities, new technology, or new staff. And the toughest staff to hire and manage are the doctors in the practice.

Is it time to add another physician or optometrist in your practice? Do current or projected patient volumes warrant the addition of more provider capacity? Let's see.

There are a number of drivers that support a decision to add one or more new providers to your practice. The most common of these is sheer patient volume, although this can be deceptive. Energetic surgeons I work with think nothing of seeing 700 patients a month. Others end the month gasping with just half of these patients. What's the right number, the figure that says, "Now is the time?" In most settings, if the average general ophthalmologist in your practice is approaching 550 or more patient visits per month (including postoperative visits) or your subspecialists are routinely transiting 450 or more visits, *and your practice is growing,* it may be time to add doctor capacity.

As you evaluate this, please be sure to examine both growth rates and the seasonality of your practice. It can be tempting to add a provider in your busiest months, only to end up with a lot of doctor down time in the quiet months. In those extreme snowbelt and sunbelt practices that are most subject to migrating retirees, do what you can to fill in the seasonal lulls with well-timed vacations or a move toward serving a younger, year-round patient base.

Also, is your practice flat or growing? A solo surgeon with a 20% annual growth rate seeing 500 patients a month now may be a little past due in starting to recruit another doctor. The same surgeon limping along with a 3% growth rate will take years to reach full capacity.

Patient demands for subspecialty care drive a significant percentage of new hiring decisions. Most general ophthalmologists start out providing comprehensive services, including services that might ordinarily be referred elsewhere out of personal interest and a lack of other patients to serve. But, with any degree of success and growth, the same surgeon years later may be able to substantiate the addition of a glaucoma, retinal, or plastics subspecialist. The best—if labor intensive—way to evaluate this is to tally internal and external service and referral patterns for several months. Doctors working semi-autonomously in a group practice are often surprised to find that the aggregate of their referrals could not only support a new subspecialist, but that the boost in cash flow supports fixed overhead, giving every established provider a substantial pay raise.

Another large influence on the addition of a provider is the need to rebalance the practice's professional team between primary, secondary, and tertiary caregivers. In most settings, it can be both financially wasteful and professionally frustrating for a cataract surgeon to be providing optometric-level care, or for a subspecialist to be providing routine medical eye care. And many high-volume LASIK surgeons would rather bring in a keen cataract surgeon than continue to dabble in an area they no longer love.

It's rarely possible to optimize individual output, but to the extent possible, techs, optometrists, general ophthalmologists, and subspecialists should all be working to their highest professional potential. If you're not doing this in your practice now, adding a provider at the right level may allow every professional in the practice to skirt burnout, work to their highest and best purpose, as well as provide better patient care.

Of course, not every new doctor hiring decision is driven by economics, or even by patient demands. Some practice owners put lifestyle and work style issues first. Here are a few examples of this:

- The surgeon who's slowly emerging physical disability obliges the addition of someone to take over their cataract cases
- The doctor who is willing and able to take a pay cut for extra vacation time off
- The small urban retinal practice with call coverage that's become too large a burden for just two doctors
- The solo doctor in their last few years of practice, who doesn't really have a large enough practice for two doctors, but who wants to pass their practice on and semi-retire

It's important to examine your practice's actual production needs, and not assume that the only option is to hire a peer. There are numerous alternatives to adding a full-time, partner-track fellow surgeon to your practice. What can you do if you do not have quite enough business to substantiate the addition of another full-time surgical provider? Here's a typical scenario: a surgeon who is seeing an abundance of clinical patients and feels they're at 120% of their personal capacity to see patients, but who is only at 50% of their desired surgical loads.

Like this common scenario, your own patient mix may suggest the addition of one or more optometrists who are easier to recruit than physicians and whose labor costs are much lower. Or you may prefer to bring aboard a medical ophthalmologist as an extender, allowing you to increase the percentage of your time spent in surgery.

Finding a part-time surgeon is getting a bit easier in some markets. About 40% of all graduating ophthalmologists are now female, and some of these new doctors are preferring to work part time for a few years while they start a family. It also seems in the last decade that new graduates of either gender are more interested in balancing life and work, which is quite feasible in today's numerous two-doctor families. In addition, I have discovered that many retirement-age surgeons who thought they could be financially free are now moonlighting to bridge diminishing returns on their savings.

Remember that another alternative to adding providers always exists: you can simply reduce the volume of patients. This is a common tactic in some urban, managed care–intensive markets, where a younger provider may establish a practice accepting all payer contracts, and then—years later—selectively drop low-paying contracts. Doctors in growing practices who decide they want to stay solo can also start limiting their practice to selected dimensions of medical and surgical eye care, referring all other patients on to compatible colleagues in the community.

Ultimately, every doctor addition to your practice will result in at least a transient dip in profits available to pay existing providers. This profit drop is readily affordable in a 10-partner practice ... not so in a solo practice, where the hiring physician's take-home income may be cut in half for a year or more. There are several ways to blunt this pay cut if yours is a smaller practice.

You can save up capital reserves before you hire. You can tap the practice's line of credit to sustain your family income, paying back the shortfall over time. But most importantly, you should make sure that your practice volume is sufficiently robust and growing so that the new doctor is busy from the outset.

Let's imagine that the facts suggest that you should indeed bring another doctor into your practice. Before actually recruiting and hiring, some additional, refined due diligence is indicated. It's critical that you examine carefully the projected financial impact of your decision. Even if there is going to be a long-term profit from adding a doctor, there is certain to be near and intermediate loss. Your administrator or accountant should draw up a *pro forma* of forecasted cash flows, taking into consideration the cost to recruit, relocate, and to cover wages and benefits, along with supplemental promotion, staff, equipment, and supplies.

Even if Dr. New is a shining star, several months may pass between their arrival (and first cost to your practice), their credentialing as a provider in local plans, and their actual generation of first collections. Still more time will pass before you'll make back the accrued backlog of on-boarding expenditures. In some settings, it can take as much as a year or longer to break even on your investment.

Few practice investments are more costly or harder to manage than adding the next doctor. Wise choices will lead to better care for patients, a larger and more harmonious team, and greater profits.

Of Happy Partners in a Group Practice

If you're an ophthalmologist, odds are high that you've learned how to work well with other people—you have to, because you serve thousands of patients a year and the odds are getting higher every year that you work in a group practice.

I'm often called in to restore doctor-to-doctor relationships in practices where the providers are no longer harmonious. Here's a checklist to improve harmony in your own setting and avoid calling in a mediator.

- *Have a written business plan.* Until the owners of a practice are clear about their goals, it's easier to have partner relationships go adrift. Your goals can be abstracted into a terse punch list or elaborated into a major document. Either way, you'll have a reference for prioritizing near-term actions and acquiring the resources you need to get ahead.
- *Employ a strong administrator.* Although no lay manager can—or should—act as a referee between arguing practice owners, the best management executives can help you keep your practice humming along well enough that there are fewer reasons for discord.
- *Select the right physician-leader.* The best practices are led by one strong lay manager and one strong physician. Too frequently, the latter is an unpaid, figurehead position only. Your group practice's MP should be elected for 2 or more years and receive a stipend that is equal to about 5% to 10% of their total professional compensation.
- *Always have a new physician-leader in the wings.* Unless your term of office exceeds 2 years, or you are pretty certain the current MP will be in place for successive terms, consider nominating the next partner who will be stepping up next. It takes at least a year or two to get ready to lead. Selecting the next leader is easier in a large practice with a deeper bench of prospects.
- *Run formal, fact-based board meetings.* It's common as practices grow to maintain the old informalities of their mom-and-pop stage. Re-read *Robert's Rules of Order* and follow them to whatever level of formality is comfortable. Your meetings will be faster, fairer, and more effective. Make decisions based on facts more than feelings.
- *Support your board's decisions. Always.* Does something like this happen in your practice: You make a decision by majority vote. Then one or more of the dissenters go out the next day and tell their staff, "I know we voted for 'X', but I'm going to do 'Y' instead—the board is wrong." Nothing will undermine overall practice morale faster than an owner who cannot respect majority decisions.
- *Pick the right doctors to join your practice.* No matter how much you interview, how much you check references, or how closely you observe their surgery tapes, only about 50% of the time will you hire the right doctor to join your practice. The other half of the time "Dr. Wonderful" will end up being "Dr. Wrong Fit." Work very hard at this and you'll be 55% correct, which will save some of the grief.

- *Remove the wrong doctors quickly.* When you pick the wrong doctor to join your practice, make your mistake as quickly as possible and find a new home for your mismatched associate. In hindsight, most hires who do not work out are visibly wrong within the first few months.
- *Oblige every owner to understand the business.* There was once a time when all you needed to know as a practice owner was the location of the key to the back office door. Not any longer, especially if you're in a complex group practice. Small errors in judgment or a lack of proper financial oversight can now balloon into a significant business killer. Rather than having just one or two doctors in a group understand the business, it's helpful to teach every owner—and also every partner-track associate—the basics of business.
- *Ensure every owner has a personal financial plan.* In the typical five-doctor client practice it's almost certain that one of the partners is mismanaging their personal financial life. This is usually due to either a lack of spending or savings discipline, which is usually linked to the absence of a personal financial planner or involved accountant. If one of your partners is making poor personal money moves, this will adversely impact their judgment in the boardroom.
- *If you need a second subspecialist, protect the first one.* Imagine you have one over-worked retinal specialist in your group. You know you need a second subspecialist. But if you add Doctor #2, you're going to hurt #1's income for 1 year or more. What should you do? The easy and fair solution is to build a floor under doctor #1's income, so that for a period of 12 to 36 months after hiring, #1's income is preserved at (let's say) 80% of historic levels. Since ***everyone*** gains over time with the addition of a new doctor, it's only fair that ***everyone*** should take the same financial hit transiently.
- *Control your practice's access to patients and share them fairly.* It's easy to control capacity—just hire a new worker or equip a new exam room. It's a lot more difficult to control the ***volume*** of the practice. Marketing, contracting, and customer service must work just right to bring you the correct mix and number of new patients. Meanwhile, make sure that the patients you do serve are shared fairly among all practice providers to preserve harmony.
- *Let doctors do their own thing ... to a point.* It's best to not unduly limit a provider's scope. For example, every appropriately trained surgeon should be able to perform cataract surgery or provide LASIK or care for patients with glaucoma, rather than only allowing the senior doctors or subspecialists do this work. But do not be shy about requiring surgeons of lower quality, despite their other abundant attributes, to give up operating.
- *Coach individual providers actively.* If you're the administrator or MP of a group practice, it's easy to focus so hard on the big picture that you forget your practice is really composed of a lot of individual professional careers. These careers should each be coaxed along at the same time that you're managing and coaching the entire team.

- *Be clear about provider productivity expectations.* Most practice overhead is fixed. If partners or associates drop off in their productivity, practice overhead goes to waste and profitability can plummet. As part of their individual contracts with the practice, providers should have reasonable volume and revenue production expectations, as well as an upper limit on time away from the practice.
- *Make the practice as profitable as possible.* As a wise old man once said, "If you think it's not about the money, then it's probably about the money." Money, as crass as it may sound, is a wonderful solvent for partner-to-partner squabbles. I've noted that partner discord is rising sharply just as profitability is declining in recent years. Do all that you reasonably can to optimize profits.
- *Share practice profits fairly.* There are hundreds of potential compensation methodologies in a group practice, and not one of them is perfectly fair over time. You need to continuously adjust and fine tune the compensation model every year or two to at least ensure that every partner is equally *unhappy* with the math.
- *Treat partner-track associates well.* Many practices are set up to treat prepartner associates as second-class citizens. Instead, provide your partners-to-be with abundant access to performance data, a voice (if not yet a vote) in management, and a robust education in the intricacies of practice ownership.
- *Hold plentiful group meetings between management and owners.* At least once a quarter there should be a time when all of a practice's owners and all management staff gather to jointly identify and solve problems. Do not leave your administrator obliged to act as postman, passing messages back and forth between the board and the managers.
- *Play together outside of the office.* The happiest group practices are those owned by doctors who not only respect their partners as surgeons and physicians, but who truly enjoy each other's company. If your practice is less "Kumbaya" than you would like, try to engineer better relationships with an annual board retreat, quarterly partner social dinners, or sporting tickets shared around the group.

• • •

The Greek philosopher Plutarch wrote (2 millennia ago) that to understand and treat in medicine one has to first examine disease. In the same manner, to understand and nourish harmony in your group practice, it's important—even if occasionally unpleasant—to face up to areas where you and your colleagues are discordant.

Of the Associate Doctor Becoming a Partner

The modern odds of hiring a partner-track physician who will actually make partner one day is dreadful and seems to be getting worse. This is frustrating for practice boards and candidates alike—and is driven by numerous errors, omissions, and false hopes on both sides of the aisle.

Only half of the time does an intended partner doctor make it to ownership. The rest of the time something gets in the way, such as:

- The young doctor fails to thrive economically, clinically, or surgically.
- There are miscommunications about the actual terms of employment or partnership.
- Interpersonal frictions arise.
- The new doctor's family does not settle well into the community.

Not all of these difficulties can be foreseen and, despite best efforts by candidate and practice alike, the odds of a fit will never approach 100%. But as a practice you can up your odds by addressing four key areas.

First, Manage Your Practice Well

Is your practice partner-worthy in today's more competitive environment? Only some of this is under your control.

If you practice in Los Angeles, and are forced to accept 80% of Medicare-allowable contracts, your practice's profit margins will never shine when compared to Midwestern clinics. But, if you can run a tighter Southern California practice than your regional peers, you will be a competitive choice for candidates who are willing to gain sunny skies for a trade-off in earnings.

If you practice in Uptown Manhattan, where ophthalmologists operate on each other to stay busy but still run a tight organization with good control over referral sources, you'll be a top pick for the best applicants.

A practice is well-run not just in profit-margin or population-per-provider terms, but also in such dimensions as:

- Existing partner cohesion—which is critically important to most applicants; after all, who wants to join a club where the members are at odds with each other?
- A positive history of prior associates making partner.
- Having a written business plan and a clearly articulated, plausible vision for the future (including, especially, a succession plan for any older, "rainmaker" members of the practice).
- Employing a strong management team, with skills deep enough in financial, IT, marketing, and regulatory dimensions to stand up to the challenges of the day.
- Providing active assistance with practice building—with direct-to-consumer marketing where indicated and internal referral support and lay staff support to make referring doctor outreach less daunting.
- Possessing, especially for subspecialists, the clinical and surgical instruments and resources needed to pursue the latest in patient care.
- Allowing providers the flexibility of crafting the professional life of their dreams, which increasingly with young candidates means working less than full time.

With these attributes, you'll be attractive to a deeper candidate pool at the front end and increase the odds of picking a potentially compatible candidate. And when the time comes for a young associate to become an owner, your relative progressiveness and business control will reduce your odds of having to start all over again.

Second, Select the Right Partner-to-Be

The six-figure investment you make in a new associate provider—much less a prospective professional peer and partner—should be undertaken with abundant caution. But it rarely is. Such hires are often undervetted and poorly consummated.

It helps to start with the cynical, but protective, premise that half of all ophthalmologist job applicants to your practice are below average. With that as a starting point:

- Generate the largest possible candidate pool; in the current competitive environment, that often means hiring one or more recruiting firms, sending out direct mail appeals to surgeons licensed in your state or region, and pestering your drug and equipment reps for leads.
- Do not settle for less than you need. If you are looking for a hard-charging, workaholic cataract surgeon who is going to take your practice to the next level, do not hire Dr. Milquetoast who wants a 32-hour-a-week job and no call.
- Beware the obvious warning signs: job hopping, equivocal reference checks with past employers, and interviewees who do not take responsibility for why their last job did not work out.
- Consider not just new grads but also mid-career providers, who have a job history you can investigate and whose maturity is likely higher than a new grad's.
- Do not make a hire until you have flown to the candidate's current setting and personally observed them in clinic and surgery.

Third, Offer Contemporary, Competitive, and Transparent Terms

Roughly 40 years ago, when I first became an advisor, training programs were increasing the number of newly minted ophthalmologists by more than 2% a year, much faster than the growth in patient demand. A newly graduated ophthalmologist was happy to get a five-figure salary and a pat on the head, with only loose promises of future ownership.

Fast-forward to today. Training programs have tapered their output to a pace resulting in essentially zero net ophthalmologist growth rates, at a time when the demand for care is growing about 4% per year and a large cohort of baby boomer ophthalmologists are heading for retirement.

As a result, the average perigraduate (or mid-career doc in a job hunt) now has several job offers to mull over. You therefore have to out-compete your fellow practices with favorable employment and partnership terms.

No more head-patting about the partnership details. Before you post your job offer you should spell out in writing (and your board should preapprove):

- Associate period employment terms (eg, base wages, bonus, benefits, work requirements)
- Future buy-in terms (ie, inclusive of the rationale for any goodwill buy-in component, which is commonly contested and has been whittled down over the years)

- Details about any finite thresholds a candidate will have to attain to be considered for partnership. (This is a commonly overlooked area, for fear of offending. As a result, an associate MD generating $500,000 in collections in their second year may silently presume they are on track for partnership, while at the same time their employers are complaining in the boardroom about their inability to thrive.)

In addition, for finalists (and increasingly commonly, their business advisors) you should be prepared to release these performance details of your practice:

- The last few years of financial statements
- Volume performance data (eg, visits, cases, referral patterns)
- The current and prospective buy-in and buy-out documents
- The story behind any recently departing associates who have not become partners
- Information on adverse conditions (eg, pending lawsuits, adverse compliance audits, contract loss)

Fourth, Actively Manage the Candidate Partner's Career

This is one of the most common practice employer flaws leading to an associate doctor's premature departure. New providers in your practice are an expensive, hard-to-replace resource. They should be actively supervised, curated, and supported. This means:

- The practice is "professionalized," that's to say, it's a serious, professional environment with every effort made to provide the best care possible. There are monthly all-hands provider meetings, giving owners and nonowners alike a chance to rub shoulders and exchange pearls.
- Reporting lines are clear. Every associate provider (eg, both partner-track and durable employees) should have a defined partner-level doctor who meets with the associate at least monthly.
- Lay staff are trained to be respectful and supportive of associate doctors. Too often, lay staff treat prepartner doctors as second-class citizens. Some of this is understandable—it's natural that a founding board member commands more respect than a 30-something newbie. But it's important that the practice's lay leaders (eg, the administrator and mid-level managers) personally demonstrate their support for partner-track providers.
- Regular performance feedback and active coaching. About quarterly, every partner-track associate should sit down with the MP and the administrator to be walked through their performance stats: cases, visits, collections, revenue and surgical densities, patient satisfaction survey results, and the like for the prior period. Throughout the initial 2- or 3-year prepartnership period, associates should be continuously aware of their prospects for ownership and any overt performance gaps.

Of Acting Like a Partner

In most professional firms besides medicine, the pool of applicants materially exceeds the number of job openings. There can be scores of great applicants for a low-level associate position in a law, architectural, or accounting firm. And even 5 years later (these are often years of 60-hour weeks), one's elevation to partnership is by no means secure.

This is quite unlike ophthalmology, where the number of open positions is growing faster than the number of available candidates and the demand for care is rising sharply.

As a result of this, some practices are lowering their guards—and their standards—by admitting partner-track associates who are unlikely to ever be partner-worthy and offering partnerships to doctors who are destined to be a poor fit.

If you have a partner-track associate heading for partnership, or even if you're only starting to interview for a new doctor, here are 12 simple screens for compatibility.

1. *Sufficient passage of time.* The prepartner associate period is typically as little as a year or as long as 5 years. The average figure in ophthalmology is 2 to 3 years. Does that figure sound familiar? It's about the same time that couples date before they seriously consider marriage. The similarities are apt. During, at least, the first year, everyone in both settings is on best behavior. But, eventually the true personality of both marital and business partnership candidates shines through (or fades to black). Beyond giving both sides time to see whether there's a fit, waiting at least a couple of years has a practical advantage—before then, it's unlikely that the new doctor has developed sufficient revenue productivity to be able to afford to start paying for a buy-in.
2. *General affability.* Pathologically unpleasant individuals, even the smartest ones, are usually screened out well before they complete an ophthalmology residency. Still, eye surgeons come in a wide array of flavors, from cuddly and affable to individuals who are described by everyone in their world this way: "Well, Dr. Andrews is not the kind of guy you go to for a good time, but he will give you a great surgical result." If affability counts in your practice (and it should), hold out for Dr. Cuddly.
3. *Clinical and judgment skills.* These are two separate skills, and both should be required of your candidate partner. Clinical skills are essential, obviously. But great didactic knowledge without the judgment to apply it properly will lead to disaster on the clinic floor. And in the courtroom.
4. *Surgical skills.* I've often asked the question, "How do you know a great surgeon is a great surgeon?" The answer that typically comes back is the same as Justice Potter Stewart's 1964 Supreme Court dictum on pornography: "I know it when I see it." And so will you, if you're judging your young colleague's fitness for partnership. Watch carefully.
5. *Compatible work ethic.* At any one time, I'm working with a large number of 60-something ophthalmologists who lament the lower work ethic of their 30-something colleagues. If you are a workaholic surgeon, it's not likely that you are going to be happy with the average new graduate's idea of a full work week. You

either need to accept that their work–life balance is going to work for you, or keep looking for the uncommon young individual today who puts their career ahead of all other life domains.

6. *Staff interaction.* One of the best partnership screens is to stay keyed into what your staff members think about Dr. New becoming a partner. If their thumbs are still up in the air after a couple of years, yours should be, too. And vice versa. If your candidate partner is humble and self-effacing, willing to drop what they are is doing to help out the crew, and someone who makes the crew proud to work as support staff in your practice, you're anointing the right candidate.
7. *Patient relationships.* Even the sweetest doctor will tote up a few patient complaints each year, especially when compared to the founder. A few complaints a month should set off alarms. A few complaints a week should lead to termination. Let your patients vote your associate in or out of partnership.
8. *Utilization and volumetric productivity.* It's helpful to pull the last year's Current Procedural Terminology (CPT) report on a candidate partner and check their utilization statistics against the average for the practice. If the existing partners have a 40% YAG rate and the junior doctor is at 15%, some comparisons around the table may be in order. The same goes for the utilization rates of special testing, assertiveness in charging for refractions, and the overall revenue yield per patient visit. Laggards should be coaxed to higher performance before they become partners. Outliers who overtreat should be counseled and if needed, removed.
9. *A well-adjusted ethical compass.* Some conservative ophthalmologists do not have the stomach for what's become of modern medical economics, where being sufficiently assertive in coding and case selection is unfortunately necessary to also make payroll and get your rent check in on time. That said, aggressiveness has to be tempered by an underlying sense of what is defensible and is absolutely in each patient's individual interest. It's a fine line and getting finer all the time. As the practice owner, you call the line. Make sure your partner-to-be is on the right side of it with you.
10. *Financial productivity.* I'm often called with a question along the lines of: "I'm the founder of a two-doctor practice. Dr. Maybe has been on staff as an associate for 3 years. His collections were $620,000 last year. Mine were $1.9 million. Is it time to bring him on as a partner?" The answer is a definite "maybe." If he passes the other screening dimensions discussed here, he could be a good fit. But since Dr. Maybe is only generating 25% of total practice collections, equal partnership may be less appropriate than a minority share of the company—or a delay in granting partnership until the two doctors are a little closer to being economic peers.
11. *Business instincts and behaviors.* When you nominate a new partner, you are not just advancing a clinical peer up the ranks—you are drafting a new board member. Each new addition to the table should ideally improve the sum total of the skill, judgment, and commitment of the board to your company. Rethink your decision if the new owner candidate is overly timid, disruptive, or absolutely disengaged from all business affairs (yet unwilling to trust and delegate business authority to others like you who are interested).

12. *Giver vs taker mentality.* As the old man used to say: There are only two kinds of people, givers and takers. Two willing givers make the best partnership. A taker can partner well with a longsuffering giver. The most toxic practice environment is a cohort of takers. Measure your candidate in black and white terms—this is not a matter of degrees. They are either a giver or a taker. Does the candidate volunteer for extra call? Cheerfully take on special projects? Or do work and worry get pushed off to others that they should personally bear? Partnering with a taker, even the most productive one, sets up the rest of your career for misery.

Of Fixing Broken Practice Boards

Practice boards, whether composed of two doctors in a modest partnership or 20, are susceptible at every turn to unresolved disagreements and unhappiness. Boards can periodically bend out of shape and many eventually "break." Like Leo Tolstoy said of unhappy families, unhappy boards are each unhappy for their own unique reasons.

Most partner-to-partner unhappiness is ultimately economic in nature, although this may be masked in more seemly terms. "I need this new laser, not just to help my segment of the practice but to keep us up with the local standard of care." "Think of the prestige our practice will enjoy if I take on this new research study." "My surgical outcomes will suffer if my packs don't contain a left-handed titanium trans-nasal retractor."

Jealousies, petty or otherwise, are a common wedge. These take many forms, including senior doctors who are jealous of up-and-coming junior partners (whom they see as having not yet paid sufficient dues). Doctors whose subspecialties limit them to more modest billings can be jealous of their more prosperous colleagues.

Conflicts can sometimes arise over a perception that there is an unfair distribution of responsibilities. A complaint could be, "As the senior partner I seem to be the only one who cares about this place. My production suffers because I spend 8 hours a week on staff problems without a word of thanks, while you all sit back and generate more income for yourselves."

Sometimes disharmony is generalized. There is no prominent disagreement, but an accretion of past hurts and controversies. "Old Shoe Syndrome" can set in and, like longtime spouses, long-term partners will progressively gnaw on each other. The cordiality and social bounds they once respected fall away, exposing pent-up hostilities. Once-close friends can no longer stand to be in the same room.

And of course, there's the human factor. Not everyone can get along with everyone else. Underlying personality issues (eg, some that are found prominently in the eye care profession: narcissism, bipolar disorder, generalized anxiety) can stand in the way of harmony. In the toughest settings, underlying interpersonal conflicts are magnified by any real or looming economic difficulty.

Board conflicts appear to be on the rise. I believe there are several reasons for this.

Most prominently, profit margins are narrowing. Abundance can paper over a lot of interpersonal conflicts. Back in the days of high fees, low competition, and 50% profit margins, it was hard for arguments about money to break out. In addition to robust personal incomes, there were very few high-ticket decisions. No six-figure computer decisions. No half-million-dollar femto quandaries.

Next, practices are getting more diverse. Intergenerational conflicts arise naturally, of course, but there's more. Twenty years ago, most eye surgeons were White, boomer-era, workaholic, 40-something males with scant work–life balance. Ophthalmology was a pretty clubby world. Today, the age, gender, ambition, and ethnicity distribution bandwidths are all much wider, which is a natural setup for more board conflicts.

Of course, practices are getting larger and more complex. This cuts several ways. Decisions are larger and harder. One wrong move can be much more expensive. The decision cycle is slower because more facts have to be gathered to come to a decision. And in large, complex practices, implementation is frustratingly slower, so problems can linger.

And finally, everyone is getting (appropriately) more anxious about the future. Even if you work in a well-run, harmonious setting today, you and your fellow owners who are projecting gloom about lower payments and higher regulatory controls naturally exacerbate shareholder frictions.

What Does a Healthy Ophthalmic Practice Board Look Like?

To recognize potential board pathology in your practice it helps to consider the hallmarks of a healthy medical practice board. Here is a list of a few:

- Wise choices are made regarding who is admitted to partnership. Economic productivity alone is not a ticket to practice ownership.
- Disruptive individuals are speedily removed from the board, and perhaps from the practice itself.
- Healthy practice boards work from well-documented governance rules, especially those rules regarding thresholds for decision making, tie-breaking mechanisms, and an appeal process for doctors who are frustrated by a board decision that did not go their way.
- Powerful, effective practices are run by powerful managing partners who have sufficient tenure and appropriate operating latitudes and who are given tough, regular feedback on their performance.
- Powerful managing partners cannot shine without competent administrators (and vice versa). Board squabbles commonly center on frustrations because the lay management team is not hitting reasonable goals.
- In harmonious board settings, we see a sufficiency—even an abundance—of meetings. For the typical practice, the board should meet monthly. The administrator should be present—sometimes with a vote, always with a strong voice.
- And last, great practices are great to the extent that they foster a culture where fearless confrontation of any open issues is the norm.

Repairing Broken Boards

While each unhappy practice board may be dissatisfied for different reasons, the path back to normalcy is analogous to a sick patient's path back to health.

First, someone on the board has to have a visceral "chief complaint"—and be sensitive and brave enough to be the first to speak up. That person needs to communicate their concerns, even if mild and still "subclinical," to other board members. For example, "Mike, I'm a little disturbed by events at our last board meeting. We normally show a lot more respect for each other's opinions, but several of us really tore into Bob. This seems to be a growing pattern. I'm afraid if this keeps up we're going to have a hard time making effective, collaborative decisions."

Next (just as in medicine) you need to seek the right kind of treatment. Some gaps in board functioning are self-resolving, like the common cold. Other gaps, wider ones, need professional help.

More group discussion alone, moderated by the board chair or practice administrator, may be enough for board members to walk back from the brink of discord. If that's not enough, you may need an expert. What kind? It depends. If you have a focused practice issue (analogous to a patient's focused clinical complaint), calling in an expert in that area may be all you need.

Let's say a board fight has been brewing about your office facility. Half of the board wants to update the building. The other half of the board wants to spare costs. Bringing in a medical space planner or architect could help to break the tie. A fresh exterior might be feasible at a lower cost than was feared (or higher cost than was hoped).

Resolving an acute, fresh, and focused controversy of recent origin can be simple. It's much tougher when positions have hardened. For these long-standing board conflicts, a different, deeper kind of facilitation may be needed:

- A forensic accountant in the case of suspected mismanagement of funds
- A trusted attorney who can help to unravel and revise outgrown shareholder agreements
- An industrial psychologist to gain insights about frank interpersonal conflicts
- A specialist billing, ASC, managed care, or similar consultant to help break a tie vote on one technical point or another

• • •

And here's a closing thought—again, analogous to medicine. Just as patients with diabetes have a chronic disease they must manage for life with good habits and ongoing medication, some boards are chronically discordant. Just as a person with Type I diabetes may need daily insulin for life, some boards need strong, regular medicine to remain healthy: extra meetings, formal leadership development, and the regular attendance of a trusted nonowner moderator to help referee meetings that would otherwise spin out of control.

CHAPTER 9

The Inner Game

It is a sad fate for a man to die too well known to everybody else, and still unknown to himself.
—Sir Francis Bacon

Of Measuring Success

Economists the world over gauge a country's forward progress and the welfare of its people by measuring gains in the GDP, defined as the total market value of goods and services produced within a given period, typically a year.

GDP growth is generally viewed as good, and the more the better. In the United States, averaging over a couple of decades, we've managed to squeeze out a bit over 3%. Until recently, China was roaring along at three times that pace in good years.

Pinto JB. *Simple: The Inner Game of Ophthalmic Practice Success, Second Edition* (pp 169-184).

Putting this in an ophthalmic context, the typical practice today is growing its collections—its GDP if you will—at about 4% per year. This coincides with the rising demand for eye care services, which should continue to be leveraged upward by the growing ranks of senior patients for at least the next 20 years.

Revenue growth is easy to measure and palpable. But a few contrary economists are advancing the concept that GDP growth and shrinkage, taken alone, are poor (perhaps even perverse) measures of national advancement or decline.

These economists have coined a new metric, the "genuine progress indicator" (GPI), to replace or supplement GDP. Wikipedia reports, "GPI is an attempt to measure whether a country's growth, increased production of goods, and expanding services have actually resulted in the improvement of the welfare or well-being of the people. ... GPI advocates claim that it can more reliably measure economic progress, as it distinguishes between worthwhile growth and uneconomic growth."

Could the same GPI concept be useful in thinking about ophthalmic economics? Even if your practice collects and generates more revenue and profit today than in the past, are you truly better off as a surgeon-owner?

Some of the happiest surgeons I know are soloists in boutique practices, who work 3 or 4 days per week, and have kept their organization small enough to be able to personally understand and have deep control over the enterprise. These doctors do not have the volumes needed to support the surgery centers, optical shops, and employed associates needed to optimize their personal income, but they ***do*** generally report a very satisfactory professional life.

Another class of happy doctors I work with are in small group practices, with two, three, or four surgeons. They keep things simple with only an office or two and well under 50 employees.

At this mid-range scale, ancillary profits from employed optometrists, optical dispensaries, and surgical facilities begin to nicely boost the personal incomes of owners without veering off into the enterprise complexity and partner frictions that can be seen in the largest practices today.

At about five ophthalmologists or more, a provider's professional satisfaction can slip, in my observation. More evenings are taken up with meetings to make decisions and solve problems. Any individual doctor loses both control over and even an understanding of how their practice works, becoming highly dependent on a few key staffers and advisors to keep the machine running.

A practice with 20 doctors instead of 1, and 200 workers instead of 10, can have more than 20 times the frequency of doctor conflicts, lay staff intrigues, regulatory near misses, and malpractice threats.

Even though practice growth, like national economic growth, is the gold standard for certifying real progress, there can be diseconomies and inefficiencies of rising scale and fast growth.

This is especially seen in selected settings:

- When a purely ophthalmic practice merges with a multispecialty medical group
- When a few small eye practices combine into one large practice
- When a dynamic MP spurs practice growth at a pace faster than doctors and staff can absorb

Well-run ophthalmology practices now measure their economic performance as diligently as countries measure their GDP. And there is plenty of agreement on what constitutes great benchmarks. But there is not yet an ophthalmic equivalent of the GPI. I believe that coming up with a GPI measure in ophthalmology is increasingly important, as now-merely-threatened fee cuts eventually come to pass, and surgeons grasp for ways to communicate with their management staff (and each other) about whether the practice is truly progressing or just racking up bigger numbers and bigger headaches.

• • •

Here's a list—in no particular order of importance—of 10 possible dimensions of your "genuine progress." How are you doing?

1. *Physician net income per hour worked.* Surely, earning $300 per hour is more satisfactory and less frustrating than earning $150 or $75 per hour. High income per unit time gives you the freedom to explore a new work–life balance, especially as you shift gears from your go-go 40s to your 50s and 60s. A low-income density may keep you on an involuntary treadmill.
2. *Sufficiency of income.* Studies have shown that a person's happiness rises with income to a point, and then plateaus. If you are not yet up to what—for you—is the necessary plateau, your sense of professional progress and satisfaction could be less than ideal.
3. *Sense of innate fairness in all partnership matters.* Compensation modeling, buy-ins, buy-outs, communication, and voice in the boardroom are just the start of a long list of partnership terms that can help an owner, in the aggregate, feel satisfied or unhappy.
4. *Change density.* Change, as researchers have learned, results in stress. This is true whether the change is something positive (eg, a new home) or negative (eg, a health setback). Too many practice changes in a year can be terribly stressful. Imagine launching a new clinical service, building a new office, converting to electronic health records, and adding two doctors all in the same year. Great progress on the surface, to be sure, but perhaps over the top in terms of your personal ability to cope.
5. *Staying at the cutting edge professionally.* This is perhaps the counterpoint of too much change density. It feels rotten to perceive that you and your practice have fallen behind the times. This includes personal and staff training, as well as access to the latest clinical tools and adoption of vanguard business systems.
6. *Intellectual satisfaction.* They do not call doctors "med heads" for nothing. Ophthalmologists thrive on learning new things and interacting with other smart people, whether these smart people wear scrubs or business suits. For some, interesting time spent solving problems with colleagues and administration can be just as rewarding as clinic or ASC time.
7. *The highest possible surgical density.* Most eye surgeons would like to see half as many clinic patients and twice as much surgery. Not only is this economically effective, but it increases professional satisfaction and accelerates surgical skills.

8. *Stable cash flows and freedom from economic or regulatory anxiety.* The practice of medicine was once quite static from generation to generation. Even as procedures changed, though at a much slower pace than today, economic sufficiency was ensured and regulations were simple to follow. We are now in an era with tapering profit margins, and with far less cushion for business, legal, or clinical misjudgments.
9. *Pleasant facilities to work in.* You spend more waking hours in your clinic than anywhere else. When you walk up to the threshold of your office, do you feel pride or pain? Are the public spaces up-to-date or shopworn? Do you personally like the art? Is your personal office a comfortable, efficient, and calming refuge?
10. *A gratifying patient base.* There is a reasonable complaint leveled by providers who are locked into serving some patient populations—noncompliant patients, HMO patients with a sense of undue entitlement in accessing your care, or snooty affluent patients. All of these can be vexing in their own way. Some of the most satisfied surgeons I work with serve high-functioning seniors and families in quaint college towns.

• • •

I'd be interested to hear from readers about this. What other dimensions of practice and career progress besides those listed previously count to you? What is their relative weighting in your own setting? Do you measure and discuss these broad elements of progress during your board and management meetings, or get bogged down in daily minutia? Would we be on a better, happier path measuring more than money and case counts in a world where these things will be increasingly rationed?

Of Excess Attachment to One's Career

Attachment is the great fabricator of illusions; reality can be attained only by someone who is detached.

—Simone Weil

The reason many people in our society are miserable, sick, and highly stressed is because of an unhealthy attachment to things they have no control over.

—Steve Maraboli

Ophthalmology is a sticky profession, with much to become attached to and much to be anxious about losing.

As an ophthalmologist today, your attachments and aversions started early. From the first days of grammar school, you ego-identified with being the smartest kid in the class and were crushed on those rare days when your class standing slipped. Not knowing the answer when the teacher called on you or bringing home a "B" on your report card generated the same motivation as a dropped nucleus does today.

Then, after 25 long years of clutching for academic mastery and performing for others—at the far end of a long, narrow tunnel—abstract knowledge became a bankable skill. The net value of your work shifted from \$8 per hour to \$8 per minute (or \$18 if you became a retinologist).

And then the real attachments began. To earnings, to fast-accumulating assets, to all the cool technology of eye care, and to the admiration of patients, peers, and the community you serve.

What we have to learn is to be free of attachment to the good experiences, and free of aversion to the negative ones.

—Sogyal Rinpoche

In a once-stable, now fast-fading, era dating from the creation of Medicare in 1965 (and yielding soon to Medicare payment reform and an increasingly creaky national economy) ophthalmologists who paid the 25-year educational toll could until recently nurture a host of attachments like these with little fear of loss:

- Keeping up your surgical skills? This was easy back in the 1980s when you only had one—maybe two—new ideas to master each year.
- Technical currency? It was easy when buying the latest gizmo was a $5,000 impulse instead of a $500,000 leap of faith.
- Retirement savings? Rock-solid and growing at a safe 12%.

Not so much now.

For those surgeon-clients nearing retirement, I routinely hear sighs of relief. They won't have to agonize over femto. They'll give electronic health records a miss. And their nest eggs are all incubated and ready to be hatched to buy lifetime annuities.

For the next younger generation of surgeons, the 30-, 40-, and 50-somethings who paid the same 25-year toll as their baby boomer colleagues and who developed the same fondness for wealth and mastery, it's going to be a different story. Their attachments to many of the superficial perquisites of the ophthalmic lifestyle—accustomed income, total control—will be stretched. And some will be ripped away.

• • •

Psychologists, mystics, and most of the world's major religious traditions counsel against the misery of unsustainable attachments. As Dr. Deepak Chopra once put it, "You are not your Toyota"—ego identification with mere things causes pain when that stuff is taken away.

As the fees paid per service unit fall in the years ahead, the healthiest surgeons will adapt. They will realize that they are not their Toyotas (or their BMWs or ski cabins for that matter). Some, in markets where hospitals will inexorably buy up specialty practices, will realize that life and the professional satisfaction that comes from serving others do not end when you move your skills into a larger institution.

Other surgeons will rail against their changing circumstances. Some are moaning now, spitting blood and nails at the injustice of disallowed fees, more documentation, new hoops to jump through, and the dawning realization that private, independent practice could largely morph to institutional practice within a generation or less.

How ***much*** will you have to adapt? Nobody knows at this point. How ***well*** will you adapt if forced to? That's the important, highly personal question that is completely under your control.

Here are four 1-day exercises that may give you some personal insights:

1. *For 1 full clinic day, set aside any thought of personal financial gain.* Practice for 1 day on a break-even basis. If you normally generate a net profit after all expenses of about $1,500 (a typical mid-range figure), write a check out in that amount at the start of the day to any favorite charity. Then do your work. Serve each patient knowing that you will get nothing, financially speaking, for it. Then sit down at the end of the day—did you feel differently about your job? Did the frank absence of a paycheck for that one day make you miserable about your work? If (like conducting a foreign mission trip) you felt somewhat invigorated giving your services away for free that day—you will be better prepared than most for what's coming down the line.
2. *For one full clinic day, practice as though you were never going to retire.* Would you arrive at the same time in the morning or a bit later, lingering over the paper or perhaps starting the day at the gym? If you were working the rest of your life, are there staff or patients you would dismiss from your practice—not really worrying about the near-term financial consequences because, hey, you're going to work the rest of your life, anyway? May as well make it fun, right? Based on this exercise, and your *actual* retirement plans, what insights do you have about how you should be practicing in the years ahead?
3. *For 1 full clinic day, practice solely as an homage to your teachers.* Begin by sitting quietly and alone for 30 minutes before the first patient arrives. Write down the names of your most influential teachers, starting with your parents and grammar school classes and continuing through to the most recent pearl you received from a colleague at a national meeting. When the first patient of the day is roomed and prepped, and as you walk in to greet them, imagine that all of the teachers you wrote down are in the room shadowing you, nodding approvingly at your work. Continue in this manner until the last patient is discharged. At the end of the day, sit down for another quiet 30 minutes and write down what you noticed about the day. How much have you advanced since your first lecture on glaucoma? Did it matter how many surgical cases you booked? Was the difficult patient a bit less irksome?
4. *Finally, practice for 1 full clinic day as though these were your last 8 hours as a physician.* Imagine that each patient encounter is your last time with that patient, and that as the afternoon wears on and the countdown proceeds until the very last visit, the sand is running out of your ophthalmic hourglass. Notice how it feels to say goodbye to each patient and perhaps how you linger a bit, or smile a bit more warmly.

• • •

Most eye surgeons attend clinic 4 days a week. Pick any week you like. Next week will do. Perform these exercises and you'll have a good read on how the rest of your career, and your life, are likely to go.

Of Provider Burnout

A little boy in the first grade goes to his mother and asks, "How come dad comes home, spends just a few minutes playing with me, has dinner with us, and then goes to his study to work the rest of the night on that briefcase of papers he always brings home? How come he doesn't spend more time with us?"

His mother leans down low, gives the boy a hug, and gently says, "Your father is a busy eye surgeon. All day long he's helping lots of people see better. He has a lot of people counting on him. So many people, that even when he's finished his office work, he still has lots more left to do. That's why we only get to see him a short time each evening."

The little boy—he's quite smart—rolls this around in his head for a moment, applies what he knows of his simple grammar school world, and with enthusiasm says, "Mom, I've got it! If dad's having such a hard time keeping up, maybe he needs extra help!"

Unfortunately, very few ophthalmic surgeons *voluntarily* slow themselves down, even when burnout looms. More often, they work full tilt and then a little harder each year until they hit the wall. This wall can be a profound, disabling physical or emotional breakdown. But more commonly, it's simply a deceleration of the rate of practice growth until a kind of equilibrium is reached where the demands of patient care and the business' complexity are balanced with an individual's ability to keep pace.

Like medieval siege warfare, your workload and stress can pin you down for years. If a surgeon's energy or attention to detail slackens even slightly more, the practice can actually spiral downward. I most often see this slow grinding burnout in solo practices and in multidoctor practices with just one owner, situations where all the responsibilities are on one person's shoulders.

In my consulting practice as a business coach to some of the country's more ambitious surgeons, I look for early signs of burnout, just like an athletic coach looks for early signs of physical injury. There's no point of increasing a surgeon's patient volumes or decreasing an athlete's marathon times if the result is an overachiever who can no longer perform at all.

Every surgeon has a different reaction to stress. Some of the country's highest-volume surgeons only get "crispy" at 300 or more major cases per month. At the other end of the scale, some anxiety-prone surgeons are like twitchy concert musicians, who can only go on stage if they premedicate for the stress induced by having to perform. Both reactions are obviously within the normal range of experience. Here are several ideas drawn from my travels around the country that may help to forestall or reverse burnout in your own setting.

- *Use diet and physical conditioning to offset mental and physical exhaustion.* Paradoxically, regular physical activity—anything from long walks to formally supervised gym workouts—can be both treatment and prophylaxis for burnout. That's perhaps why we see that some of the nation's busiest surgeons are extremely fit physically. It may help to enlist the help of a personal trainer and a dietician to start a program if you need an external source of discipline.

- *Increase delegation.* You don't personally have to do everything. Have your optometrist or senior tech take first call, with you available for standby. If you're in solo practice, take on a junior partner or recruit an administrator with enough sophistication to take the business worries off your plate.
- *Decrease your cost of living.* Many surgeons slip unconsciously into a pattern of increasing the cost of their lifestyle just slightly faster than their hard work can keep up. The stress of excess debt and a spouse asking when the family's second home can be redecorated—on top of an already stressful practice—can put even the most burnout-resistant doctor over the top. If necessary, enlist your accountant or hire a financial planner to help you adopt a personal budget that's chronically 20% to 50% less than your net after-tax practice earnings.
- *Reengineer or eliminate the unnecessary.* Not *everything* needs to be done. If you have a surgery center and you're burdened by residual hospital duties, draw back to courtesy status if this is politically feasible. Are you writing letters when a quick call or an email message will do? Shift gears and communicate in the most streamlined way possible. If you dictate at the end of the day, shift to dictating in front of the patient at the end of the encounter—it really does take less time (since you're already oriented right then to the case) and it's working smarter because you save steps in discussing the treatment plan with the patient. Learn to say "No" to responsibilities that do not make a proportional contribution to your business. You might want to still chair an annual vision screening program in your community, but decline speaking once again during career day at the local high school. Any of the many recent books on simplifying your life may help you commit to an undercommitted lifestyle.
- *Establish boundaries.* Are you like the doctor in the previous story, with a satchel of paperwork to plow through each night? Consider setting boundaries. Even small steps like: "I do not EVER work Wednesday evenings, which are reserved for family night," can be remarkably liberating. Use your appointment calendar not only to be disciplined about when you're available to see patients, but when you're not available at all.
- *Change the duration and periodicity of time off.* The typical eye surgeon takes about 4 to 6 weeks off a year. Half of this is commonly spent at national meetings. Granted, the meeting locations are often posh, but such meetings are hardly a break from the office. Indeed, by the time you factor in the added stress of travel, worries about leaving the office uncovered, and the anxiety at hearing about how many LASIK cases your old roommate Charlie is now doing can all add up to returning home more stressed than when you left.

  Examine yourself closely and adjust the frequency and duration of time off. For some clients, taking a long weekend twice a month is more rejuvenating than 2-week vacations—and can actually result in far less down time away from the practice. At the very least, if you must combine vacations and continuing education, arrive a few days early to enjoy the meeting city with no responsibilities. Rather than trying to hit every meeting every year, rotate among the meetings and order audio recordings for any important sessions you simply can't miss.

- *Slow down.* We can learn a lot from surgeons who, as they enter their 50s and 60s and become financially independent, start working a schedule that pleases them. Surprisingly, they rarely quit. Instead, they transition to 3- or 4-day weeks. They refer the toughest cases. They develop deeper relationships with a few pet patients and favorite staff members. If you're in your 30s or 40s, taking this approach early may grind the sharp edges off the least pleasant dimensions of your practice.

• • •

Note that many of the previous approaches to stress reduction may have an almost inevitable adverse impact on profitability. This does not have to have a proportional impact on physician take-home pay. Indeed, the last thrashing efforts to get ahead can, in some settings, yield diminishing returns. An increasing number of clients who were once striving to cross their finish line to economic freedom well before traditional retirement age are now realizing there's nothing they like better than working. Since slowing down and eliminating the least pleasant aspects of their practice, they'll happily work a little longer and end up with just as much financial security as if they had burned themselves out trying to reach a premature finish line. As you may have already experienced, a 5% decrease in your clinical or surgical schedule can have a 50% increase in your work life quality.

Of Career Satisfaction

Much of modern ophthalmic practice is as sweet as it was 50 years ago. Helping patients in need. Proving meaningful employment and coaching for support staff. That delicious nexus of intellectual and manual mastery.

And then there's the rest of it. The "muck of practice life," as a dear mentor of mine puts it.

Unfortunately, the "sweet-to-muck" ratio is diminishing for many surgeons today. Paradoxically, those in larger group practices, where external pressures can conflate with internal partner-to-partner frictions, seem to have the fastest-falling ratios today I see as I travel around the country on assignment.

• • •

Several years ago I developed a tool to sort through the many variables that go into providers' satisfaction with their current professional situation.

First, you and your colleagues around the boardroom can use the results of this tool to learn more about each other, which is the start of a more intimate and effective team of owners. When I'm working with a dispirited board, one of the root causes is a lack of sufficient understanding of—and empathy for—each partner's priorities. This is pretty fundamental stuff. What are you looking for as part of a group practice setting? What's important to you? Are you getting it here?

Second, this tool may help you put your finger on what's bugging you most about your present practice situation and see it in context. If there is something you rank highly as a desired aspect of practice, and the score is particularly low, this item will fall into sharp relief and force you to think about what you can do to make improvements in that area.

And third, I hope that even if you don't use this as a board exercise (or if your "board" is YOU alone) that you will take this tool for a test drive and gain some personal insights about how good you really have it on balance, despite the mucky bits.

Read each of the following 13 items. After each, enter an A, B, or C score for how important this item is to you, and a number between 1 (low/terrible) and 10 (high/wonderful) to rate how satisfied you are about that dimension of your practice life.

For example, for item 3 below asking you to rank and rate ***community***, you might write down an "A" (because where you live is very important to you) and a "9" because (because you really enjoy where you live).

Pinto's Physician Satisfaction Rank and Rate

1. *The initial associate employment terms.* If you are still an associate of the practice, are the terms fair, reasonable, and contemporary? Are the rules logical and positing in a way that improves patient care and practice success (even if they may inconvenience you personally)?
   ____ Rank (A, B, C)
   ____ Rate (1 to 10)
2. *The partnership buy-in cost and terms.* If you still have not bought in (or have done so recently), is the pricing fair and in line with similar opportunities around the country?
   ____ Rank (A, B, C)
   ____ Rate (1 to 10)
3. *The community one lives in.* Do you and your family have access to desired amenities, scenery, culture, recreation, your spouse's career opportunities, child education options, etc?
   ____ Rank (A, B, C)
   ____ Rate (1 to 10)
4. *Peer-to-peer relationships.* Is your practice characterized by professional harmony and the absence of conflict? Or, do one or more doctors in the practice make it unpleasant to come to work?
   ____ Rank (A, B, C)
   ____ Rate (1 to 10)
5. *Support staff.* Are lay staff competent? Do they receive sufficient oversight and development by management? Do day-to-day working relationships contribute or detract from your job satisfaction?
   ____ Rank (A, B, C)
   ____ Rate (1 to 10)

6. *Access to needed resources.* Do you have a reasonable measure of the staff, facilities, technology, practice-building promotion, and other resources needed to thrive?
   ____ Rank (A, B, C)
   ____ Rate (1 to 10)
7. *Control over your access to patients.* Are new patients fairly apportioned between doctors? Do senior doctors do their part in passing along patients or do junior providers have to hustle and compete to build their own practice segments?
   ____ Rank (A, B, C)
   ____ Rate (1 to 10)
8. *Independence.* Do you have the ability to practice your profession without unnecessary oversight or control from above (while of course yielding to appropriate group standards)?
   ____ Rank (A, B, C)
   ____ Rate (1 to 10)
9. *A fair voice in policy and governance.* Are you allowed to participate to an appropriate degree in business and medical policy decisions? Are you kept "in the loop"?
   ____ Rank (A, B, C)
   ____ Rate (1 to 10)
10. *Compensation.* Is the provider comp methodology—and your personal income level—equitable, proportionate to effort, and in line with market rates?
    ____ Rank (A, B, C)
    ____ Rate (1 to 10)
11. *Bonding and attachment to a cause greater than oneself.* In healthy group practice settings, the ***collaborative*** delivery of superior eye care can provide a significant source of career and life satisfaction, as well as feelings of pride, security, solidarity, team belonging, etc. How does your practice measure up?
    ____ Rank (A, B, C)
    ____ Rate (1 to 10)
12. *Durability/sustainability.* Do you have a sense that all the favorable variables will remain the same or improve in the years ahead?
    ____ Rank (A, B, C)
    ____ Rate (1 to 10)
13. *Exit strategy.* Is there a sense of fair pricing and terms for doctors (including you!) as they leave the practice?
    ____ Rank (A, B, C)
    ____ Rate (1 to 10)

After completing your rank and rate for these 13 general items, feel free to add any other dimensions not covered in this list that make your professional life satisfying and meaningful. For you, career satisfaction may be the ability to take a mid-day exercise break, teach at the local university, or have hours flexible enough to take care of young children.

Finally, ask yourself these questions:

- Based on insights gained from completing this exercise, what's my overall level of satisfaction with my current professional setting?
- Are the items that are most important to me scoring highly?
- Is there one hot button item that I need to address acutely, or do I have mediocre feeling across several different categories?
- Is it possible for me to make improvements in these scores?
- Can I make these improvements on my own, or do I need help from peers, managers, or outside facilitators?
- Are improvements feasible in this practice, or only possible if I leave and start somewhere else?

Of Security

When I was growing up in the 1950s and 1960s, the atomic threat was front page news. In grammar school we were subjected to monthly duck-and-cover exercises. I can still remember vividly the grainy 16-mm civil defense film clips demonstrating a proper "duck" and Miss Short, my third grade teacher, admonishing us to be sure to lace our fingers tightly behind our necks so the soon-to-be-flying shards of glass wouldn't sever our impressionable young heads.

Some of the crankier and more paranoid folks in my Los Angeles neighborhood actually started digging bomb shelters and buying up a 3-year supply of powdered eggs. All things considered, the more sensible of us kids thought at the time that the adults were being a little crazy. And anyway, instant vaporization would probably be preferable to being locked up in a hole with your parents until the radiation fell to safe levels.

• • •

Fast forward to today. All of the adults are ***still*** running around in a panic. Perfectly sensible surgeons and managers and lobbyists and congresspersons, each in a lather over a highly unlikely but nonetheless nuclear fee-cutting blast from Washington. The only things missing are the do-it-yourself Geiger counters and those eerie air raid sirens.

Still, it *c-o-u-l-d* happen, this Medicare fee-cut bomb. So, an abundance of caution is not entirely unreasonable. What would a proper level of caution and defensive preparation look like under the circumstances? Duck-and-cover drills probably won't cut it—your administrator will still find you hiding under your desk and bring you the latest Centers for Medicare & Medicaid Services (CMS) news release from Washington. And these days, an underground shelter is better for your Bordeaux collection than for hiding out from this month's cliffhanger fee-cutting bulletin.

Something more practical and robust is needed in the typical practice, and something more suited to calming your spirits than your body. You need something that lets you KNOW you will be able to survive whatever comes out this year, or next year, or the year after.

So here it is. Pinto's Patented Practice Medicare Bomb Proofing List—6 simple mental drills. Pin this list to your office wall. Read it out loud every time that scary email surfaces.

1. *Know your own truth.* You are one of only 15,000 MDs in America who are trained and licensed to cure eye disease and prevent blindness. You are smart, resourceful, and you possess a degree of animal cunning, with self-preservation instincts borne of MCATs, 36-hour work shifts, your toxic second-year neurobiology professor, and possibly divorce attorneys. If you have to, if your back is against the wall, you can work longer, faster, and harder than anyone else you have ever met.
2. *Know the promising truth of the eye care profession.* The demand for your services is rising 4% per year now. And the baby boomer tsunami is just starting to roll into the beach. The number of ophthalmologists has flatlined. (While the US population has grown about 11% in the last decade, the number of residency slots has shrunk about 11%.) This is great math, anyway you slice it.
3. *Remember: You are mobile.* If you work in an overdoctored city, you can move to the country (to rural America), where eye surgeons are scarce and practice expenses are scant. You would in short order have a robust practice, low lifestyle costs, and plenty of money left over at the end of the month to fly your personal plane back to the city on weekends. With the right choice in markets, and a little extra work, make that a personal jet.
4. *Really, really mobile.* If things became truly dire, you could pack up, leave America, find a job in lots of pleasant corners of the world, and earn a top 1% income just as you do now. Do you feel it's impossible to consider pulling up roots? Think of this Medicare mitigation strategy as simply a well-paid, long-lasting mission trip, and you'll be just fine. (And you'll leave your American colleagues in an even better bargaining position, with one less competitor.)
5. *You are not an island.* If there ever is a thermonuclear Medicare fee cut that sticks, the ***entire*** health care world will shift on its axis. Private payer fees are ultimately indexed to Medicare rates. There would be an abrupt downdraft in payments to all ambulatory care providers and a pretext (and the pricing power) for you to apply a comparably abrupt cut to all inputs: lay staff labor costs, facility rents, capital equipment. God forbid, consultants, too. The works.
6. *You will still be happy, no matter how much fees are cut.* Studies of human happiness indicate that after the first $100,000 or so, with the essentials of life covered plus a few niceties, we do not get happier making more money.

• • •

In another 50 years, we can hope that today's Medicare's serial cliffhangers will seem as quaint and anachronistic as the nuclear scaremongering of the last century. All the same, it's nice to know how to dig and duck, if only to work off a little nervous energy.

Of Retirement

A few times a year I get a call that goes something like this:

Caller: You've got to help us out. We've got a big problem in our practice.

Me: What's the problem?

Caller: It's our senior partner, Dr. Ed.

Me: What's he done that's so bad?

Caller: He promised he would retire at 68, and he has just turned 74.

Every single ophthalmic career without exception, including yours, will transit a predictably parabolic arc though five stages of varying lengths:

1. Your professional life's birth when you are about 30 years old
2. Growth and development as you learned the inner game
3. Maturity and hopefully a nice, long run of it
4. Decline and senescence
5. And finally, professional death—occurring for some in their 50s, for most in their 60s, and for a lucky few in their 70s or later

Given baby boomer demographics and shrinking residency training slots, about 40% of America's ophthalmologists are 55 and older. That percentage will climb in the next 15 years.

Because eye care is such an alluring field—and not a particularly physically demanding one, unlike orthopedics—ophthalmologists have always retired somewhat later than the US average of 62. My typical male client retires late in his 60s (despite firm assertions in his 50s of a retirement in "about 5 years").

This general shift to older retirement, once entirely driven by the pleasures of the profession, has been leveraged sharply upward in the last few years by the Great Recession of 2008, by the pandemic, and by ongoing challenges to practice profitability. Retirement nests are missing a few eggs of late, and lower/riskier investment earnings are projected for many years ahead. At the same time, active income from practicing has tapered off even for even the hardest working eye surgeon.

I predict that for many, 72 will become the new 62. Which all means I'm going to be getting more calls like the one discussed in the beginning of this section.

Some surgeons who work late in life show no signs of slowing down. When the beloved emeritus surgeon Dr. Herve Byron was late in his 70s, his handshake was crushing and his mental faculties were as sharp as a graduate student's. But not every surgeon enjoys Byronesque genes.

So, what's the right age for a surgeon to retire, and how should this delicate issue be handled in your practice?

There is a mandatory retirement age of 56 for air traffic controllers. Commercial pilots can stay on the job until they're 65 in most companies. Catholic priests and bishops are edged out between 70 and 75. And of course, the Pope gets to go all the way to the end of the line.

This issue should be examined from both sides of the boardroom in your practice, from the perspective of both the periretirement surgeon and their juniors.

Most older surgeons I have worked with through the years have been understandably conflicted as retirement approached. Paying your training dues and becoming a surgeon buys 30+ years of respect, control, financial abundance, intellectual challenge, and a sense of worth and purpose. That's hard stuff to look at through the rearview mirror, especially at a time when it's becoming much harder to predict future investment earnings and inflation rates.

Younger surgeons at the board table are also commonly conflicted in their feelings. If the senior doctor leaves, there ***will*** be more work and income left behind for the junior partners. But on the other hand, the doctors who remain may have to buy out the retiring surgeon for hundreds of thousands of dollars. Some patients may leave. There will be one less revenue producer to help cover fixed overhead. Perhaps the senior doctor has been a rainmaker, stimulating referrals as well as maintaining institutional relationships and securing managed care contracts.

Here are six targeted recommendations in this sphere to reduce conflicts:

1. *Put it in writing.* Your group practice's operating agreements should spell out at least a first approximate mandatory retirement age—that is, the age at which the board, without undue hand wringing, can dismiss a partner-surgeon or curtail their scope of practice. Ideally, the clinical and surgical competence of each provider (eg, MDs and ODs, partners and nonpartners, young and old) is reviewed periodically and impartially. Superior practices do not just intervene when there are gross competency gaps but help the entire professional staff elevate the quality of care each passing year. Fair surgeons can become good ones, and good ones great.
2. *Put your cards on the table.* If you are a senior member of your practice you should tell your partners as precisely as you can when you plan to retire and invite their feedback. Describe in as much detail as you can, not only the date, but the trajectory. "I would like to stop surgery in 2 years, work 2 days per week, and retire fully at 68." If you are a younger surgeon, do not shy away from discussing your anxiety about your older colleague's career plans, in either direction—speak up if you think their early ***or*** late departure will harm the practice.
3. *Monitor performance.* When is it time to stop operating? Stop seeing clinic patients? Thoughtful solo surgeons at every age and stage should have a couple of trusted colleague-mentors who they can continue to learn from and, when the time is ripe, can periodically give an honest assessment of the senior doctor's competency. This process is easier in large group practices, where a standing quality assurance committee should be in place.
4. *Make retirement a professional decision, not a financial one.* At any one time, I am working with a number of surgeons who wish they could retire but are unable to because of a financial reversal. To the extent possible, plan your career and your personal affairs so that you are financially independent many years before the earliest age at which you can conceive of actually retiring. The happiest surgeons I know are those who are over their financial finish lines at 55, but who intend to work until 65 or older.

5. *Give yourself options.* Let's say you're 45 years old now and contemplate working until you are 60. Those 15 years will go by fast. You can expect that you will change your mind and decide to practice longer. Until your actual retirement date is within close sight, you should behave in your professional life as though you are still in the early years of a vibrant career. Keep up your reading, continuing education work, and meetings. Learn at least one new clinical or surgical maneuver each year. Stay technically current. Leave the door open for a much longer career lifespan than you currently contemplate.
6. *Mediate, do not litigate, through difficulties.* As financial pressures mount, more surgeons will be obliged to overstay their welcome in their group practice. I've seen every imaginable practice conflict in this area. Make sure that your operating agreements spell out a fair, fast, inexpensive third-party process—both for protecting the rights of surgeons who want to linger and for curtailing or removing a partner who needs to go.

• • •

While he did not mention anything about vacation homes or golf outings, Sir Francis Bacon counseled that one's advancing years work out best with an abundance of just four things: old wood to burn, old wine to drink, old friends to trust, and old authors to read. I hope you live the rest of your years in abundance, helped in some small way by the concepts learned in these pages.

Afterword

A Psychologist's Perspective on the Inner Game of Ophthalmology

The only really interesting thing is what happens between two people in a room.
—Sir Francis Bacon

This is an attempt to polish just a single facet of this comprehensive gem of a book. Speaking as a psychologist, and at the risk of driving home a bit too forcefully some things you might have already learned from reading this book, these are the ***inner game*** keys to your success:

- Knowing how to better understand and respond to the sometimes subtle personal power dynamics in any group, whether you are a leader or a follower
- Knowing how to further advance your personal sensitivities and people skills, regardless of where you are in your career development

Attaining world-class results in the highly complex, fast-changing health care landscape requires a marathoner's heart: sustained, arduous effort. Massive

Pinto JB. *Simple: The Inner Game of Ophthalmic Practice Success, Second Edition* (pp 185-187).

self-discipline. Mental toughness and persistence. With a fervent, contagious passion and an optimism that your efforts will succeed.

Absent these qualities, MPs drop out of the race. Administrators collapse well before the finish line. Their fellow providers and staff suffer along the way.

It's About the Energy and Hope You Bring to a Dream

Whether working as a low-level staffer or as an owner-surgeon, mustering and sustaining a high level of psychological and emotional energy is a prerequisite for success. Such energy can only arise through the experience of *hope,* the most valuable and mission-critical asset of any practice.

Hope is naturally provoked when we experience two necessary conditions that are insufficient alone: *dreams* that have personal meaning and importance and *confidence* in the possibility that such dreams might eventually become reality.

The most compelling, inspiring, and unifying practice dreams always serve a purpose greater than you as an individual. Yes, you are certainly working hard to achieve a good income and the respect of patients and peers, but don't do so at a cost to the greater public good that you are serving, ***which is to enhance the quality of life for those in your community.***

Ultimately, in world-class practices of any size, from solo to institutional, greatness only comes on the heels of a culture committed to such a selfless dream.

Relationships Are Everything

Every business, especially ophthalmology, is ultimately driven by people interacting with other people. The key moving parts in your practice are not slit lamps and lasers, but doctors, patients, support staff, vendors, colleagues, and payers.

Our relationships drive not only our success or failure, but also determine whether we enjoy the journey. Its only human nature to resist that which we resent, which explains why spirit-deadening relationships in practices with poor morale, conflict, and interpersonal strife ultimately lead to business failure, even if on the surface the "numbers" are strong.

The foundational inner game of long-term practice success is building great relationships at every level, including with fellow owners and board members, your entire staff (and in some cases, their families), your patients and their loved ones, local colleagues (and competitors), outside vendors, and third-party payer representatives. All of these are part of a wide web of relationships. You know your web is functioning highly when the relationships are mutually empowering in healthy ways, when you feel empowered and supported by others, and then feel naturally inclined to reciprocate.

Power and responsibility must be proportionate. Power obliges responsibility, at every level of your practice. Surgeons are not permitted to operate unless they have formally proven themselves to be trained and responsible. Administrators, though less formally trained than doctors, generally progress through a career spanning ever-greater responsibility, until they have proven themselves worthy of directing a multi-million-dollar company and making decisions affecting scores of families and tens of thousands of patients.

Please consider these closing, inner game concepts:

- Encourage everyone in your charge to be just as productive and result-oriented for the greater good of the patients and the overall practice as they are for the owners and themselves.
- Accordingly, emphasize teamwork and loyalty, first to each other, then to the job—since you can't accomplish the results without working in a durably aligned manner.
- Serve the men and women under you first... by teaching, coaching, and advocating for them as their champion; giving them a voice; and doing everything to help them get what they reasonably need.
- However, you also serve those men and women under your supervision by not necessarily giving them what they ***want*** and by confronting any inappropriate or mission-threatening behavior. Remember that *what we don't confront, we enable.*
- Remember that each of us is connected interdependently—we need each other. The power and loyalty you enjoy as a leader flows directly from the power and loyalty that you give to those under you.
- Make it your priority to be consistently trustworthy, through your demonstrated competence as well as your good character, diligence, and promise-keeping.

• • •

Make it your regular practice of self-improvement to answer these questions, including seeking input from trusted staff and peers when you are not sure of the answers:

- Am I an accountable servant leader, humbly serving a mission greater than myself—or do I impress others as being primarily concerned about my own welfare and prosperity?
- Do I demonstrate a leadership style in which others feel empowered, valued, appreciated, and encouraged to find and express their voice—or do I show more of a dictatorial approach?
- When I become frustrated, anxious, irritable, or tired, do I take responsibility for my interaction with others, shielding them from my moods—or do I expect others to adopt to my adverse behaviors and change in order to improve my temperament?

—*Craig N. Piso, PhD*
Wilkes-Barre, Pennsylvania

Craig N. Piso, PhD is the founder and president of Piso and Associates, LLC, an organizational development consulting firm based in Northeastern Pennsylvania. Dr. Piso is a Pennsylvania-licensed psychologist with training and experience since 1979 that has included family systems clinical practice, corporate managed behavioral health, and consultation within health care, business, and education. He is an author, contributing to numerous books and periodicals, and he is an award-winning presenter at diverse professional development conferences. Craig can be reached at (570) 239-3114 or cpiso@pisoandassociates.com.

Last Word

Pinto's Ten Commandments

By far the best proof is experience.
—Sir Francis Bacon

We all, even the hardest working among us, like things really, really simple. For all our lofty ambitions, there's something about the soaring human spirit that doesn't want to work too hard… that loves a distilled list of dictums for improvement.

Thus, the best-selling self-help books promise the reader that perfection is just a few enumerated steps away (ie, always in 10 or fewer steps, as you may have noticed), as in:

- *Three Steps to Permanent Fat Loss*
- *Five Steps to Lasting Financial Freedom*
- *Seven Steps to Finding Durable Love on the Internet*

Pinto JB. *Simple: The Inner Game of Ophthalmic Practice Success, Second Edition* (pp 189-192).

There are the *original* Ten Commandments, of course—which stretch the upper 10-point ceiling of convenient enumeration and memory. And then there are "Pinto's Ten Commandments" that, at the risk of being both too derivative and too profane, I developed many years ago in response to a time-poor client who asked for the *Cliff Notes* version of practice enhancement.

It's always been tough to build and keep a great practice. Indeed, half of all practices are below average in profits, in growth pace, and in control over operations. It's so much tougher to be above average now, leaning into the headwinds of health reform.

This is as good a time as any to haul out the tablets once again, with apologies to Moses, and be reminded of a few simple rules that can put you—and keep you—at the top of the pack.

Pinto's Ten Commandments

1. *Hire the best people you can afford and treat them right.* Beyond your own brains, training, and ambition, your support staff are your practice's most valuable business asset. How well is this asset growing in value? Arrange things so that every new hire you make, as well as every staff termination, improves the aggregate performance of your human resources. Remember that keeping staff performance and morale high is more a matter of how well they are treated than how well they are compensated. Memories are long; we have an almost perfect recall of how others make us feel.
2. *Provide staff with 1 hour of education for every 79 hours of work.* This doesn't sound like much time, and it's not. It is only about 1% of total payroll costs, by the time you factor in benefits costs. But very few practices actually hit this profit-enhancing standard. This has always been a mystery, given that every physician who signs a payroll check can be counted among the most educated people in human history. You know from personal experience the value and the payback of training. You've spent the largest single block of your life as a student. Apply this fundamental truth to creating a continuously smarter organization.
3. *Keep tomorrow's appointment book 100% full.* Do you have the kind of staff who let out a sigh of relief when the clinic schedule is light? Serving just one extra patient per day can increase annual profits by $35,000 or more. Try this little experiment: Tell your entire staff that for 1 week you're going to be running a "full capacity" test in the practice. The goal is to fill 100% of the available template, less the inevitable ± 5% no-show rate. As a reward at the end of each day for hitting this goal, tell staff they'll each receive a crisp, new $20 bill. (Or, if you want to limit costs, just reward the reception staff who are directly responsible for keeping the template full.) If your experience with this test is in line with others, you and your staff will learn that it really is possible to look ahead in the template and backfill any holes.
4. *Treat every patient as though they were your only customer.* I learned this from a mentor many years ago when I hung my consultant's shingle. Still works in any line of business. Fake yourself out and try it during your next clinic session. Not only will your patients notice a difference, but so too will your staff, who will work to match your elevated customer service standards.

5. *Ask every patient to refer a friend, every time.* Although it may feel a bit weird, even profoundly uncomfortable for the first few days, following this pearl can boost your new patient volumes by 20% or more. And, it will cost nothing but a few moments of your time. Deliver the following, simple words to each departing patient in the spirit of a public health message, while also handing them three of your cards: "Please tell your friends about the importance of regular eye care." Ninety-nine percent of your patients will smile back at you. Ignore the 1% who snap back with something like, "Oh sure, doc, so I can wait twice as long to get in to see you next time." This gets easier the longer you do it, and a lot more effective if you follow Commandment #4 and give them something to rave about to their friends.
6. *Know your numbers—cold.* To become a physician you mastered thousands of normative physiological benchmarks. In a way that is probably still very intellectually gratifying, you know how the human machine works and how it occasionally breaks down. You know the right diagnosis and the right treatment plan because you can measure health and sickness by the numbers. The same is true in running a business. Happily, the structure and function of your practice business can be mastered and monitored by knowing fewer than 100 normative benchmarks. Think through business problems like a doctor—by knowing your numbers cold—and you'll build a great practice.
7. *Find a surgeon more competent than you and copy what they do.* There is only one best cataract surgeon in the world, only one best LASIK surgeon, one best retinologist. So, the chances are extremely high that you have something more to learn. Find a clinical or surgical mentor and learn what they know. Then pass it on to someone down the ladder from you.
8. *Sweat every detail, even the ones that bore you.* Remember, we all like it simple and easy. Therefore, this commandment is one of the toughest. Kind of like the "thou shall not covet" of the business world. Here's a prominent example. If you own a mid-size or smaller practice—let's say one with fewer than five fellow doctors—you need to be personally, technically conversant with your billing system and protocols. You should be able to audit a chart for adequate documentation, post a charge, submit a clean claim, run reports, and interpret a host of patient accounts metrics. Owners of larger practices are generally off the hook with this particular commandment—you have a fleet of management executives, who in turn direct an armada of technical specialists to tend to the myriad details of the practice. (Think about that the next time you get to drive home early, leaving your administrator behind to solve the problem.)
9. *Remember, financial success is measured in profit per hour, not cases per month.* Chest-pounding about your high personal case volumes may be satisfying, until your more efficient local competitor drives circles around you and your high overhead practice. As a general ophthalmologist working in today's environment, your pretax income should be about $150 or higher per hour worked—in a practice with a 35+% profit margin—with the ability to comfortably see 40+ patient visits per day. If you're not hitting these numbers or higher, it's time to learn how before the next phase of health reform changes the norms… and your income.

10. *Live on less than 80% of your after-tax income and invest the rest intelligently.* Even if your personal resources are relatively unbounded, you and your spouse should develop and live within a budget that allows for adequate savings rates. Unfortunately, if you only start living by this commandment late in your career, or if you pursue foolish investment risks, you may have to learn how to live on less than 50% if you want a comfortable retirement. So it goes.

• • •

Will these 10 commandments guarantee you a wildly profitable, enjoyable practice? Inner peace? The amazed admiration of all those around you? No. Especially not in these interesting times. For that, there's the eleventh commandment, adhered to by the happiest surgeons I know:

11. *Have fun ... let go a bit. .. get into trouble a bit.* Be content and just a little less than perfect when circumstances allow. Enjoy the moment-by-moment of your practice and your life, rather than dreading some unborn future. Be mindful of and grateful for your abundant life. Give freely of your miraculous skills to those in true need. Remember that your professional career is ultimately among the most secure on the planet. There is, and will always be, an unlimited and chronically underserved market demand for not going blind.

Index

For Product Safety Concerns and Information please contact our EU representative GPSR@taylorandfrancis.com
Taylor & Francis Verlag GmbH, Kaufingerstraße 24, 80331 München, Germany

www.ingramcontent.com/pod-product-compliance
Ingram Content Group UK Ltd.
Pitfield, Milton Keynes, MK11 3LW, UK
UKHW021957180926
475701UK00003B/70

* 9 7 8 1 6 3 0 9 1 9 5 9 7 *